Sex, Lies,

and the

Truth About

Uterine Fibroids

Sex, Lies,
and the
Truth About
Uterine Fibroids

A Journey from

Diagnosis to Treatment to

Renewed Good Health

Carla Dionne

Avery

A MEMBER OF PENGUIN PUTNAM INC.

NEW YORK

Most Avery books are available at special quantity discounts for bulk purchase for sales promotions, premiums, fund-raising, and educational needs. Special books or book excerpts also can be created to fit specific needs. For details, write Putnam Special Markets, 375 Hudson Street, New York, NY 10014.

a member of
Penguin Putnam Inc.
375 Hudson Street
New York, NY 10014
www.penguinputnam.com

Library of Congress Cataloging-in-Publication Data
Dionne, Carla.
Sex, lies, and the truth about uterine fibroids : a journey from diagnosis to
treatment to renewed good health / Carla Dionne.
p.   cm
Includes bibliographical references and index.
ISBN 1-58333-070-4
1. Uterine fibroids—Popular works.   I. Sex, lies, and the truth about uterine fibroids.   II. Title.

RC280.U8 D55   2001   00-066397
616.99'366—dc21

Printed in the United States of America
1   3   5   7   9   10   8   6   4   2

Book design by Patrice Sheridan

Illustrations designed by
Natalie Gallmeier (Uterus, Fibroid Uterus, and Anastomoses)
Carole Raschella (Men Survey cartoon)
Melissa Dionne (Cyberspace graphics)

Acknowledgments

Without the support and love of my husband, Richard, and three children—Melissa, Alex, and Brian—this book would never have been written. My love and thank-you go out first and foremost to these four individuals who never left my heart at any time while I was writing. I love you guys. *And yes, Brian, NOW we can go to that theme park you've been bugging me about!*

Special thanks to Jean P. Curtin, a librarian who responded to my endless requests for research. Librarians are the salt of the earth and the best people to have around you when you have questions that demand answers based in research. You're the best, Jean. ☺

Many other individuals frequently came to my assistance with information, guidance, medical insight, and support. I can't say enough about Scott C. Goodwin, M.D., and Michael S. Broder, M.D.; both were kind and generous in giving me their time and responding to a multitude of email with medical questions.

Thank you also to each and every physician, health professional, and patient advocate who shared their knowledge and thoughts on a wide variety of subjects related to uterine fibroids and the variety of conditions that women suffer through with this disease. Special thanks to all the following: Tori Hudson, Jennifer Berman, Laura Berman, William Parker, Herbert Goldfarb, James Spies, Robert Andrews, Robert Worthington-Kirsch, Steve Smith, Anne Roberts, Wendy Landow, Beth Tiner, Elizabeth Plourde, Lise Cloutier-Steele, Marsha Weaver, Leonie Finkel, Thomas

Lyons, Eric Schaff, John Thomas, Francis Hutchins, Marian Mizokami, and Dora Skalisky. The variety of in-person, telephone, or email conversations held with each of these individuals helped me tremendously in shaping the information presented in this book. Sometimes, the simple act of expressing support was enough to keep me going on this project. I can't thank these people enough nor can I begin to list all the additional individuals who contributed to this process as well.

Quite a few years ago I was fortunate enough to be receiving medical care from a physician who taught me that doctors are fully capable of talking *with* their patients and empowering them with knowledge so that, as a team, the patient and physician could make medical decisions *together*. He's been the yardstick that I've measured all of my subsequent physicians against and a tough act to follow. Thank you, Peter Bours. You have no idea how much the simple act of providing an open, patient-physician communication environment meant to me. Indeed, communication that empowers is the very foundation of this book.

Finally, thank you to all the women on the Internet who opened my eyes and made me realize that I was truly not alone. Your sharing and your support have meant the world to me. Cyberspace. Who would have ever thought it would mean this much to so many women? Care to join us?

For my father . . . a man who taught me to question what is real, what is right, and what is "just" in this world . . . a restless vagabond soul who searched his entire life for the path to what is true and found the answers to his deepest questions at the end of a fishing line on the riverbanks of the Snake River. I miss you Dad.

Contents

Foreword

Twenty-five percent of women in the United States will have symptomatic uterine fibroids in their lifetimes. Despite the prevelance of this disease, very little is known about what actually causes it. In addition, the medical therapies are only palliative and the only permanently curative surgical procedure is hysterectomy, which entails removal of the entire diseased organ. Of the 600,000 hysterectomies performed annually in the United States, over 200,000 are performed because of uterine fibroid disease. Per capita, these numbers are far larger than for any other Western nation. Many authors have expressed concern about the size of these numbers and have discussed the personal, political, social, and economic issues that sometimes come into play when decisions are made regarding patient care. One publication concludes that 70 percent of hysterectomies are performed inappropriately. In recent years, because of the number of women with symptomatic fibroid disease who often undergo hysterectomy, there has been a push by many investigators toward developing less invasive alternatives. These include watch and wait, hormonal therapy of various kinds, myomectomy, myolysis, and uterine artery embolization.

I was largely unaware of the issues surrounding hysterectomy until 1996. It was in that year that we started offering uterine artery embolization for the treatment of uterine fibroids to women in the United States. Embolization, which is the introduction of a substance into a blood vessel to stop bleeding or to treat abnormal blood vessels or tumors, has been performed worldwide for more than three decades. In this procedure an interventional radiologist introduces a small plastic tube or catheter into the blood vessel or vessels supplying the abnormality and then makes a picture of these vessels and the abnormality by injecting contrast, also known as x-ray dye. The physician then can inject a multitude of different substances as circumstances require to block these blood vessels. Embolization in the pelvis to stop bleeding after surgery or after childbirth has been available for more than two decades. In the early 1990s, an obstetrician/gynecologist in Paris, France, named Dr. Jacques Ravina noticed that patients who had undergone embolization either preoperatively or to treat bleeding secondary to fibroids subsequently had shrinkage of their fibroids and improvement of their symptoms. He and his group started offering uterine artery embolization as a primary therapy for the treatment of symptomatic uterine fibroids. They first reported their results in the English literature in *Lancet* in 1995. We presented our preliminary results in 1997, and the response by the media and by the women in this country was unbelievable. This response reaffirmed the message that alternatives to hysterectomy are needed. Much also needs to be done to better understand the disease processes that have frequently led to hysterectomy. In addition, more needs to be done to educate women about their own bodies and about all the various alternatives to treat diseases unique to women. I have been amazed and disappointed at the number of women I have spoken to who have been told they needed hysterectomy and who had not been told by their physicians about a single available alternative. Of course, many physicians believe that it is their job to decide what is best for the patient and then offer only that single option. This is not a philosophy that I personally ascribe to. I believe our job as physicians is to help the patient understand the disease they have and to make them aware of all of their options and let them make a truly informed decision.

One of the women who made a decision about her own health care was the author of this book, Carla Dionne. As you will read in these pages, she underwent a uterine artery embolization for the treatment of symptomatic fibroids. Since having undergone the procedure, she has been a powerful force in helping women to understand their bodies and learn about their health care options. She goes into detail about the epidemiology, etiology, and diagnosis of uterine fibroids in the early chapters in the book. She then goes on to a thorough discussion of all available treatment options for a woman with symptomatic uterine fibroids. There are also excellent discussions of the psychosocial and sexual-function aspects of uterine fibroid disease and also of the various treatment alternatives. A large amount of material is presented about the various information resources available to women. I know because of the scope of this book that it will help many patients. I hope it will help many physicians as well. Physicians should never forget that patients are people, that diseases are tragedies, and that patients should be fully informed, active participants in their care.

Scott Goodwin, M.D.
Chief, Vascular and Interventional Radiology
UCLA Medical Center
Department of Radiological Sciences
Los Angeles, California

On Over-operating in Gynaecology

Shortly afterward came a brief but not very creditable period when "clitoridectomy" was strongly advocated as a remedy for numerous ills. This fortunately had a very limited currency and was speedily abandoned.

Then followed a time in which displacement of the uterus held the field, and every backache, every pelvic discomfort, every general neurosis was attributed to mechanical causes, and must needs be treated by uterine pessaries. Again, we had an epoch when oophorectomy or castration of women was not only recommended and largely practised, as a means of restraining haemorrhage in bleeding fibroids, but also as a remedy for certain forms of neurosis even when the ovaries were healthy or not seriously diseased.

Ere long it was discovered that removing the ovaries for neuroses, even if safely accomplished so far as life was concerned, besides unsexing the woman, was frequently followed by more severe nervous penalties than those for which it had been used as a remedy; that, in fact, it often entailed a loss of mental equilibrium, and sometimes ended in insanity. . . .

A too reckless attempt at progress not only impairs the reputation of gynaecology, but the experience and recognition of faults must be gained

The above text was originally presented and published in 1895; subsequently, it was published as an excerpt in the *British Medical Journal* 1995; 311: 593. It is reproduced here by permission of the BMJ.

at the expense of much suffering to many patients—patients of the gentler sex, on whom no man with a spark of chivalrous feeling would desire to inflict unnecessary pain. They are absolutely at the mercy of the medical men, and submit in blind faith to what he recommends as the best to be done under the circumstances. . . . The first instinct should be to try if an operation can be avoided, not to seek reasons for performing it. **[BMJ] 1895; ii:284**

Sex, Lies,

and the

Truth About

Uterine Fibroids

Introduction

Uterine fibroids symptomatically affect approximately one in four women in the United States. Many are immediately directed down the hysterectomy path by their gynecologists. They are never told that there are other choices and decisions to be made. As a result, hysterectomy is the second most performed surgical procedure in the United States today. For women, it is the number-one most performed surgical procedure.

An estimated 600,000 hysterectomies are performed every year in the United States. In the last twenty years, over 12 million women in the United States have undergone hysterectomy. Out of those 12 million, roughly 177,000 to 366,000* were performed annually for the treatment of uterine fibroids. Those numbers add up to between *3.5 and 7.3 million women* in the United States over the last twenty years who have undergone hysterectomy for a relatively benign disease.

Despite those incredibly high numbers, there are even more women who are unhappy with the recommendation for a hysterectomy who choose to simply ignore their doctor and their physical problems—that is, until their bodies and uterine fibroid symptoms *force* them to "do something." Then they begin a long and difficult walk down the road to researching their options and determining whether or not there is a more

* Statistics vary depending upon the institute collating the data, the researchers reviewing that data, and their criteria for inclusion. Hospital discharge records from select institutes have shown an average of 45 percent of all hysterectomies performed are based on the admitting diagnosis of uterine fibroids.

agreeable solution that they can comfortably and safely choose. Sometimes they simply find themselves reluctantly and unhappily "giving up" and "giving in" to the hysterectomy option. Sometimes they choose to continue suffering instead.

Women who are diagnosed with uterine fibroids experience a numerous variety of physical conditions and stages. No two women develop uterine fibroids in the same manner, at the same pace, or with the exact same combination of resulting symptoms. Although millions of women in the United States are walking around with uterine fibroids, we are all different. As a result, we all react to the diagnosis differently and, **based on the information provided to us by our physicians,** we make the best decisions that we possibly can.

Over fifteen years ago I was diagnosed with uterine fibroids. Initially startled by my doctor's diagnosis (I was twenty-eight years old at the time), I was relieved to hear from her that it was "nothing to worry about" and that I could simply "ignore them." Not the complete truth, exactly. Not an intentional "lie" either. A mere blurring of the details. I left the doctor's office that day with little to no information about my uterine fibroids. She reassured me repeatedly that there was simply nothing to worry about and, therefore, I didn't need any additional information. Considering what I was told in that office visit, how could I have ever known that there would be much more to come in the following years?

After several years had gone by, my fibroids began causing a great deal of bleeding. They could no longer be "ignored." When I returned to my doctor, I was informed that it was time for a hysterectomy. Huh? How did it come to *this?* From "nothing to worry about" to "hysterectomy" in only a few short years. I was in shock. I left the doctor's office in complete silence, engulfed with disbelief and fear of what lay ahead for me. By the time I had put the key in the ignition of my car, I was crying. How did any of this happen? *Why me?*

On my drive home from my gynecologist, I noticed a rather large bookstore. I did a U-turn, pulled in, and purchased every book the store carried on the topics of uterine fibroids, hysterectomy, and women's health. I read every word in every book I purchased. Then, I cried even more.

The tears didn't stop the bleeding or the growth of the uterine fibroids. I knew that *something* had to be done. So, based on everything I read, I started with the simplest quick fix available. I modified my diet. The results were amazing. A few simple dietary changes brought the abnormal bleeding under control and bought me a few more years without surgery.

Meanwhile, the fibroids continued to grow and, eventually, the heavy bleeding returned. Along with it came a tremendous amount of lower back pain. I pulled out my research and reviewed my options again and decided that a myomectomy—a surgical procedure that removes only the uterine fibroids and not the uterus—would be a good choice for me. I did not want a hysterectomy. The long list of potential complications that can occur with a hysterectomy terrified me. In addition, the thought of losing my uterus and, potentially, some aspects of my sexual response concerned me a great deal. Finally, ovarian failure and the potential requirement for hormone replacement therapy did not thrill me. No. I did not want a hysterectomy.

After over a dozen consultations with gynecologists and an equal number of recommendations for a hysterectomy—not a single doctor would agree to do a myomectomy—I almost gave up. **Almost.** I simply did not want a hysterectomy and nothing could clear my thinking on that subject enough to allow me to submit to surgery that would remove my uterus. Anger borne out of the conversations I had with gynecologists fueled me to endure my fibroids a little longer and dig a little deeper for a better answer.

Eventually, my uterus and fibroids grew to the size of a six-to-seven-month pregnancy. Big. Really big. HUGE. My life was miserable, my body was wracked with pain, anemia (from passing large blood clots each month during my period) drove me to bed nightly by 7 P.M., and I knew that something, anything, had to be done soon.

By now, thirteen years had gone by since my initial diagnosis. In returning to the bookstore I discovered that not many new books had been written on the subject of uterine fibroids. So, I purchased a personal computer, subscribed to an Internet Service Provider (ISP), and quickly discovered that the World Wide Web had exploded with information. I decided to start from the beginning using this new research tool as my guide.

I was amazed and overwhelmed with the quantity of information available. It took me months to sort it all out. When I was done, I decided that other women needed an easier way to access the information. An Internet website called *Sex, Lies, and Uterine Fibroids* was born. This book is based on my experience and the initial information found at that website but also includes research gathered from medical literature written by doctors from all over the world and, subsequently, interviews with many of those doctors. It's also based on the thousands upon thousands of email, postal service mail, and phone calls from women suffering with uterine fibroids that I received after placing the website online.

During the last year, the title of this website has been a subject of some controversy. It's important to explain that it was never my intent to proclaim that all gynecologists "lie" to their patients. In fact, when I placed the word *lies* in the title, it was meant to reflect that a lack of complete communication about all currently available treatment options and potential side effects is, in fact, often viewed by the patient as a "lie." Withholding information, for whatever reason a physician may give, is frequently the foundation for miscommunication and ultimate distrust that a patient may have for her physician. Indeed, research has shown that communication is a critical factor in the patient-physician relationship. Communication (or lack thereof) has been strongly correlated to patient satisfaction, health outcomes, and even malpractice litigation.

Many gynecologists have written to tell me that they don't "lie" to their patients and express anger and dismay over the title of the website. Many other physicians have written to tell me that they know of gynecologists who do, in fact, deliberately "lie" to their patients in order to convince them of the necessity of a hysterectomy. Oddly enough, after one million visitors to my website and thousands of email, not a single woman sent me even so much as one email taking exception to the title. Not a one. But a great many of them understood the title deeply, describing firsthand experiences that clearly demonstrated the concept of miscommunication, incomplete information sharing, lack of informed consent, and the relationship of all of those to the word *lies* in the title.

Do physicians lie to their patients? Some do. Most don't. Some aren't aware that incomplete information is construed as a "lie" by their patients. Some simply don't keep up-to-date on the latest medical information and can't, therefore, communicate current treatment options to their patients that they don't know about. Ultimately, communication is the key to maintaining a strong patient-physician relationship and the foundation for whether or not a patient implicitly trusts her physician and the information that is shared.

All the material in this book proved useful to me during my search for an answer to my fibroid situation. However, I do not, necessarily, endorse or support all the ideas or research contained in this book. In fact, there is information provided in this book that is thoroughly disgusting to me. Nonetheless, it is extremely important to me that each woman decide for herself what to believe, endorse, and follow. It is equally vital for each woman to discuss with her physician whatever material intrigues her (as a possible solution to her uterine fibroid condition).

This book is divided into nine chapters and models the process by which most women begin their search for answers. Chapters 1 and 2, *Why Me?* and *Anatomy of a Fibroid,* address how doctors determine the presence of uterine fibroids, who gets them, the physical aspects of fibroid tumors, and continued research as to why they develop. In addition, I describe many of the different kinds of diagnostic tests that doctors choose to perform in analyzing and treating a woman's uterine fibroids.

Chapters 3 through 6 contain a detailed review of all currently available choices for treatment of both the *symptoms that result from uterine fibroids* and the treatment options that are used to *treat the fibroids* themselves. A recent study published in **Obstetrics and Gynecology** titled "The Appropriateness of Recommendations for Hysterectomy" determined that as many as 70 percent of hysterectomies performed were recommended inappropriately and that roughly 76 percent did not even meet the hysterectomy guidelines set by the American College of Obstetricians and Gynecologists. Although the *Treat the Fibroids* chapter does give you the latest information about your hysterectomy options, all these chapters combined lay out a road map of appropriate steps you can take and alternative options available to you that may help you avoid a hysterectomy altogether.

In recent years there have been many advances in treatment options, but one option in particular shows rather exciting results along with tremendous success stories: *uterine artery embolization.* As this is a relatively new procedure, every attempt has been made to include the latest-breaking information available from interviews with leading interventional radiologists and gynecologists.

Chapter 7, *Related Health Issues,* takes a look at many of the interrelated health problems that may or may not be present as part of a woman's overall condition along with her uterine fibroids. Oftentimes, other aspects of a woman's health are looked at as separate items by doctors and treated as though there were no relationship to uterine fibroids at all. However, each of these related health issues, if present, contributes to the overall decision that a woman makes when determining what her "true" choices are for the treatment of the uterine fibroids.

Chapter 8, *Making a Decision,* goes straight to the heart of actually making a decision. It discusses doctors (how to find a good one!), the issue of "informed consent," and the kind of information your doctor should be willing to share with you. It also covers insurance concerns, and the influence and pressure that come from family and friends. Oftentimes a woman can make a decision that may feel right for her, but no one else lends the support she needs. Many factors influence the final course of treatment that a woman actually receives. This chapter touches upon the factors that carry the most weight.

Chapter 9, *Keeping a Journal,* discusses the importance of keeping a personal journal of medical events. It specifically addresses how and why you might want to make notes of conversations and information presented to you by doctors. In addition, it shows you how to keep track of all ongoing personal-health issues. Although not entirely necessary, this type of medical tracking may prove beneficial to you and your doctors in understanding, caring for, and treating your uterine fibroids. I've included a sample of my own journal pages that has proven extremely helpful to doctors in my care and treatment.

In addition to the valuable resource information provided in this book, I have tried to share frank accounts of my own situation and thoughts as they unfurled during the research process. These are further supported by a wide variety of thoughts and feelings from other women who chose to share their experience with uterine fibroids with me.

Luckily for me, by the time I began my research through the Internet, enough time had passed that several new and promising treatment options had become available for uterine fibroids. Ultimately, I chose Uterine Artery Embolizaton (UAE)—now called *Uterine Fibroid Embolization (UFE)*—for treatment of my uterine fibroids. While this was MY choice, YOUR choice needs to fit *your* circumstances, overall health, and beliefs.

If you are a woman diagnosed with uterine fibroids, you may identify with some of the information and stories presented here. Ultimately, this book was written for you to arm you with knowledge, to make you aware of your choices, to empower you during the decision-making process, and to remind you that **you are not alone.**

If you are a supportive spouse or significant other to a woman experiencing uterine fibroids, perhaps the information provided in this book will help you to better understand the depth of experiences and choices that your partner is confronting.

If you are a physician, perhaps you will recognize yourself somewhere in this text and make whatever adjustments are appropriate in the way in which you inform and treat your female patients.

It took me a long time to realize that I was not alone in my search for answers to this health problem. Believe me, you are not alone either. Remember, somewhere around 25 percent of all women in the United States develop symptomatic uterine fibroids during their lifetime. I wish each and every one of you the best of all available choices and experiences, a supportive network of family and friends, and positive relationships with physicians who genuinely care about your health and long-term well-being.

Carla Dionne
carla@uterinefibroids.com
http://www.uterinefibroids.com

One

Why Me?

I don't know why I got stuck with uterine fibroids. I wish I did. Since uterine fibroids are benign masses growing from the uterus and not cancerous at all, you'd think they'd be easy to deal with and a cinch for doctors to treat. They're not.

Over the years that I've had to put up with my tumors, one thing has become very clear to me: fibroids suck. Okay. I know I can state the situation better than that and possibly even use a word that doesn't offend people. But, the truth is simple—they suck the life right out of you. They start out small, but if they're left unattended they can end by enlarging your uterus to the size of a basketball. Yes, a basketball. If you prefer fruity comparisons—like many gynecologists—you can take your pick from the produce section . . . orange, grapefruit, cantaloupe, honeydew, or watermelon. A fibroid-laden uterus can and does get as large as a watermelon in some women. Uterine fibroids can take a normal, approximately six-ounce, pear-shaped uterus and turn it into fruit salad that feels as though it weighs a ton and is uncomfortable, at best. In the process, fibroids can:

- divert mass quantities of oxygenated blood to your uterus.
- increase your incidence of headaches . . . most likely migraines.
- bring on severe menstrual cramps.
- create massive blood loss during your monthly menstrual period and every other day of the month.

- press your bladder into action every thirty minutes or so requiring a constant stakeout of rest rooms wherever you go.
- turn you into an exhausted, anemic rag doll.
- make you look pregnant all the time. (*Boy, did I get tired of people asking me when the baby was due!*)
- help you to *develop* your fat cells.
- pull your back muscles out.
- press on pelvic nerves.
- cut off circulation to your legs.
- damage other internal organs.
- make childbearing difficult, if not impossible.
- ruin your sex life.
- bring on severe bouts of PMS.

The PMS brought on with fibroids is not "normal" premenstrual syndrome. It's a direct result of **estrogen-run-amok** or, quite possibly, **progesterone-nowhere-to-be-seen,** and it's from way beyond the degree of moodiness or depression many women without symptomatic fibroids experience. Who wouldn't have PMS with a list like this? It gives me PMS just reading the list!

The items identified on the above list were from **my** *short* list. Every woman with uterine fibroids is different and every woman has her own *short* list. If you're reading this book because you have fibroids, I bet you can easily sit down and put together a short list of your own.

So. **Why me?** That's a question that is surprisingly difficult to answer. When I first began to research my condition, one of my doctors gave me the following list of risk factors for fibroids printed in a handy-dandy pamphlet:

- obesity
- diabetes
- stress
- smoking
- sedentary lifestyle

I didn't buy it, and you shouldn't either. I was never obese until *after* I developed fibroids. I'm not a diabetic. I don't smoke. I used to bicycle twenty miles a day (before fibroids). We *all* have stress. While I've met women with fibroids who fit *some* of this profile, I've met *more* women who simply don't.

Did the uterine fibroids develop because of my "health style"—or, did the "health style" develop as a result of the uterine fibroids? None of the current explanations for the development of fibroids has been solidly founded in research. In fact, many of the "risk" factors one generally sees listed as having an association with uterine fibroids don't typically occur until AFTER a woman has developed fibroids.

An even bigger question that is, apparently, even more difficult to answer is: Can anyone explain where in the world hormones fit into this whole picture? What triggers hormonal malfunctioning that leads to symptomatic fibroids in some women but not others? *All in all, I would really like to know just one thing: Why **did** my hormones start running amok without my permission???* Now **that** is the million-dollar question. Right next to: *If the why is known, can the treatment for prevention be somewhere close by?*

You see, where uterine fibroids and research are concerned, my guess is as good as yours. Even though doctors have known and written about uterine fibroids for over 150 years, little has been done in the way of research that would advance our knowledge of the whys and wherefores of this disease.

So What DO We Know about Uterine Fibroids?

I don't know where my doctor got his information to put together that handy-dandy risk factors pamphlet, but I do know that much of it is either inaccurate or misleading in how it was presented to me. Let's go through the list item by item and then address what researchers really DO know about uterine fibroids to date.

First item on the list: obesity. While obesity has been *associated* with the presence of uterine fibroids—it hasn't actually been determined to *cause* uterine fibroids. It's a chicken-or-egg sort of deal. There's definitely a relationship—but what is it? Some researchers believe that hormonal imbalances between progesterone and estrogen occur in a woman's body that may, very well, alter her metabolism. When this occurs, fat cells develop that are capable of storing excess quantities of estrogen. In turn, this excess of estrogen stored in the body can contribute to the development and growth of uterine fibroids. Of course, not all women who develop uterine fibroids are overweight. This complicates the picture in terms of determining the role of obesity in uterine fibroids.

Second item on the list: diabetes. I haven't been able to substantiate any correlation whatsoever between diabetes and uterine fibroids. Why was it on my doctor's list? I can't answer that for sure. From talking and writing to women all around the world, I've discovered that many unsubstantiated items make it onto a doctor's list of risk factors for uterine fibroids. Often this is a direct result of the specific doctor's patient population. In other words, it's extremely possible that the doctor who put together the pamphlet I received noticed a significant number of patients who were diabetic and who also had uterine fibroids *within his practice*. That doesn't mean it's a true and validated risk factor. It only means that one doctor noticed this trend within his practice. (We'll address this again in chapter 6, *Treat the Fibroids*—where you'll see how important this issue of physician/patient population can be when it comes to the way doctors present treatment options to their patients.)

Stress. A number of books have been published addressing stress and its relationship to the growth of uterine fibroids. None of it is research based. Not an ounce. Of course, after one learns she has uterine fibroids, stress certainly might start kicking in, particularly when the gynecologist starts telling you that you may need a hysterectomy. It certainly caused me stress where none had existed previously!

Endocrinologists do believe that *chronic* stress can cause your body's hormonal signals to get confused and result in progesterone and estrogen levels getting knocked out of balance. Dr. John R. Lee is one physician who addresses this topic at length in his book, *What Your Doctor May NOT Tell You about Premenopause.*

There's certainly nothing wrong with trying to reduce the amount of stress in your life to bring everything back into balance. It is doubtful, however, that doing so will have any bearing whatsoever on the growth (or shrinkage) of your uterine fibroids. *If you have a hormonal imbalance that is contributing to the growth of uterine fibroids, the hormonal imbalance needs to be treated. Once fibroids have developed and are symptomatically increasing in size, simply alleviating chronic stress is an insufficient remedy for treating the hormonal imbalance or the uterine fibroids and has little impact at this late stage of the game.*

Smoking. Now here's a risk factor where there has been conclusive research that clearly indicates smoking has a correlation to *reduced* incidence of uterine fibroids. Because smoking causes arteriosclerosis (hardening of the arteries), any blood flow to fibroids would be somewhat strangulated and definitely hindered from feeding the tumors. Don't get me wrong on this issue, though. I'm not saying that women who smoke DON'T have fibroids. Many do. I'm also not saying you should take up smoking to constrict those blood vessels and stop the fibroids from growing further! Smoking, as most of us are well aware, certainly contributes to a wide variety of health risks. I'm just saying that it's not a risk factor that has been associated with *causing* fibroids. Quite the contrary.

Sedentary lifestyle. Oh boy. Another chicken-and-egg sort of risk factor. Fibroids definitely slow a woman down. Are doctors really making timely and appropriate connections tying risk factors such as "sedentary lifestyle" to uterine fibroids? Probably not. They may see a correlation—but they honestly can't make a determination as to when those associative risk factors kicked in. Before or after the growth of the fibroids? Not a single research study has been done that would answer this question.

Show Me the Research!

So why do as many as one-fourth or more of all women get fibroids? Why me and why you?

First of all, let's back up a little. While around 25 percent of all women will have fibroids that cause troublesome symptoms, the actual number of women who have fibroids is probably closer to 80 percent. That's right. Four out of five women have fibroids. The majority of fibroids remains small—less than 1 centimeter in diameter—and do not cause any problems at all. Generally, they are only discovered after death and during an autopsy. Most women are not even aware that they have uterine fibroids.

If fibroids *are* going to cause problems, they generally do so when a woman is between the ages of thirty-five and forty-nine. While it is still unknown as to why, African-Americans are twice as likely to have fibroids as Caucasians or Asians. (African-Americans also end up having hysterectomies two to three times more often.) Women who have never carried a child to full term have a slightly increased risk of fibroids and, finally, oral contraceptive use does *not* seem to have any correlation to increased risk of symptomatic fibroids. These are the items that are known to have some kind of relationship to symptomatic uterine fibroids.

Although research has been slow in getting off the ground as far as uterine fibroids are concerned, it does seem to have finally piqued the interest of some scientists, and it's about time! Some additional factors that have been uncovered are:

- Fibroids have abnormal chromosomes.
- Each fibroid is derived from a single cell and related only unto itself with each additional fibroid that grows also being derived from a unique single cell.
- Changes in a woman's hormone levels may have an impact on fibroid growth.
- Fibroids grow rapidly during pregnancy when hormone levels are elevated.
- Fibroids shrink after menopause when hormone levels are decreased.
- Estrogen and progesterone play a role in fibroid growth.
- Consumption of red meat is associated with the presence of fibroids.
- Consumption of leafy, green vegetables is associated with the absence of fibroids.

As you can read, the list of what we know about what causes uterine fibroids to grow and ultimately become symptomatic is short and doesn't provide us with many real answers. We have a very long way to go before a solution to this disease is found. In the meantime, hundreds of thousands of women in the United States seek out and desperately need treatment for their symptomatic fibroids every year. There isn't, however, a miracle cure for uterine fibroids and there won't be until we know for certain what causes them in the first place.

Why me? I honestly don't know—but it was most likely a combination of many different factors, a multitude of factors that combine differently in every woman and cause each one of us to develop fibroids differently and experience symptoms differently. It's highly unlikely that any two women would have the same answer to this question.

Two

Anatomy of a Fibroid

Bet you never thought you'd be back in biology class again trying to understand basic anatomy this up close and personal, huh? Well, you can always call it a day and simply trust your doctor and not ask any more questions about your fibroids, but I cannot overstress the importance of learning all you possibly can about your condition. I encourage you to dig in and learn a little bit more about your body and what, exactly, is happening inside you. There's nothing wrong with trusting your doctor and working *with* him on a solution to your fibroid problems while you're *also* learning everything you can about your fibroid situation. That way, if and when the time comes to make a choice about treatment, you can do so confidently, with your eyes wide open and, with more complete knowledge of your body and your options.

What Is a Normal Uterus?

A woman's body is truly an amazing machine with the reproductive system always running in the background like a finely tuned engine built with, it is hoped, only the best parts. For years doctors have been writing about hormones and their interaction with the entire reproductive system. Often, the female reproductive system is referred to as a "symphony" with perhaps the ovaries representing the "conductor" of the orchestra. It has also been referred to as a finely "choreographed" movement that can become ugly and an almost unbearable performance to watch when any "dance" element (ovaries, uterus, cervix) is removed. To get a better understanding of what the "proper" functioning of the reproductive system is and why doctors have referred to it in so many interesting ways, it's important that you also have a basic understanding of the **Uterus** and all its relevant components.

A "normal" uterus is typically the size and shape of an upside-down pear and weighs somewhere around 6 ounces. Its dimensional size is about 8 to 10 centimeters by 6 centimeters (roughly 3 to 4 inches by 2½ inches). Who would have ever thought something so small could become so controversial in the medical community and bring about such incredible physical problems for so many women?

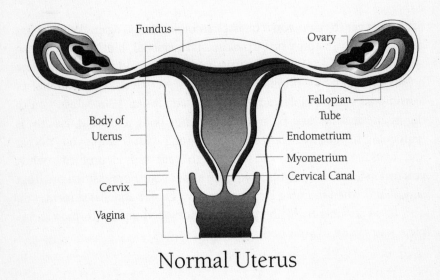

Normal Uterus

Body of Uterus Normal site of implantation of fertilized eggs
Cervical Canal Area from vagina through the cervix to the body of the uterus
Cervix The lower portion of the uterus
Endometrium The lining of the uterus
Fallopian Tube Tube that eggs travel through when they move from the ovary to the uterus

Fundus The top of the uterus; the area between the fallopian tubes
Myometrium Muscular wall of the uterus
Ovary Organ that contains eggs and produces hormones
Vagina (Birth Canal) Area or passage from the uterus to the genitals

Although these look like pretty simple body parts located roughly in the vicinity of your lower abdomen, the real truth is that they are much more complicated than they appear. On top of that, your ovaries, your central nervous system, and a couple of areas in your brain called the hypothalamus and pituitary gland run your entire hormonal cycle.

The hypothalamus produces gonadotropin-releasing hormones (GnRH), which in turn control the release of two other hormones in the pituitary gland—luteinizing hormone (LH) and follicle-stimulating hormone (FSH). These two hormones subsequently control a woman's entire reproductive cycle. In the first half of your menstrual cycle, FSH stimulates the ovaries to produce estrogen and in the second half LH kicks in to stimulate the production of progesterone. Basically, the hormones your body produces affect the entire production of estrogen in your ovaries as well as the growth of your endometrium that occurs each month.

Estrogen then circularly affects your overall continuing release of hormones in the hypothalamus, pituitary gland, and central nervous system. Estrogen also brings on ovulation (release of eggs) and affects both the uterus and vagina—and, ultimately, the growth of uterine fibroids. All in all, it's an extremely delicate balance among your ovaries, your central nervous system, and hypothalamus and pituitary gland. Any disruption to this balance can create a bit of chaos. Perimenopause is a prime example. As your hormones start fluctuating in your mid to late forties, symptoms such as hot flashes, insomnia, fatigue, irritability, depression, and difficulty concentrating are all common. Most of these symptoms settle down after menopause when hormones stop fluctuating on a daily and monthly basis.

Prior to menopause, is it any wonder that when the "battery" (your reproductive system) develops "corrosive materials" (polyps or possibly cysts) or you "take out a gasket" (uterus, cervix, ovaries) and don't replace it with anything that the engine doesn't run nearly as smoothly as it did previously?

Throw in an extra fibroid or two as a result of the balance of hormones going haywire and you'll quickly understand why most women with fibroids suffer from "running out of gas"—anemia or fatigue. In addition to that, most women I know who have undergone surgical removal of their ovaries (oophorectomy) certainly have problems with overheating.

Note: *Please forgive my comparisons of the female reproductive system with a car engine. I thought it important to come up with a comparison that both women **and** men could understand, particularly since more and more men are getting involved in the health care of the women they love. Reading about "symphonies" was meaningless to my husband. But give him a car—hey, a smoothly running engine he can understand!*

What Is a Uterine Fibroid?

Leiomyoma. Fibromyoma. Fibroma. Myofibroma. Myoma. Tumor. Fibroid Tumor. Uterine Fibroid. *A thorn by any other name is still a thorn.*

Uterine fibroids are solid pelvic tumors of the uterus. Generally, they develop out of the myometrium and are smooth muscle matter. Noncancerous. Composed of a wide variety of cellular materials and fibrous tissue. Known to have a "whorled" appearance that spirals or is circular in nature.

Just a Thought

As I wrote this section describing uterine fibroids, it kind of struck me that I was detailing some sort of criminal pattern—sort of like what a detective might do on a crime scene. Uterine fibroids are nothing more than thieves deciding to move in and stay awhile—sucking your life away, making a mess of things, and stealing precious time that could be better spent on enjoying your life. The real crime, however, is that we simply don't have a cure yet.

There are three primary types of fibroids: submucosal, intramural, and subserosal. Submucosal fibroids grow and protrude into the endometrial cavity and usually cause heavy bleeding. Intramural fibroids are located within the myometrium or uterine wall and can also cause abnormal menstrual bleeding, pelvic pain, back pain, and some pressure. Subserosal fibroids grow from the serosal surface (outer portion) of the uterus and do not, in general, cause abnormal bleeding unless they grow unusually large and press inward on the uterus. Subserosal fibroids can, however, cause pelvic and back pain along with pelvic pressure.

In addition to those three types of fibroids, submucosal and subserosal fibroids can also be pedunculated. This means that they grow off of a stalk and hang a bit separately from the uterus. Pedunculated submucosal fibroids grow from the endometrium and hang down into the uterine cavity from a thin stalk. Pedunculated subserosal fibroids hang off of the serosa, or outer layer of the uterus, also from a thin stalk. Fibroids that are attached to the uterus by a stalk may twist and turn—sometimes causing pain, nausea, or fever.

In very rare cases, cervical fibroids can also develop.

The majority of all tumors are intramural or subserosal and are actually hybrids and not just one "pure" type of fibroid at all. Only 5 percent of fibroids are submucosal.

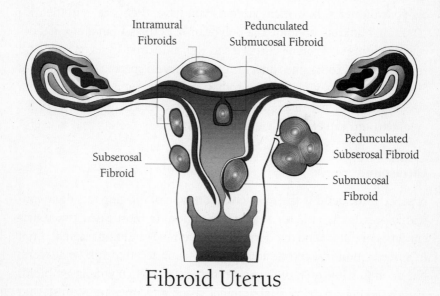

Intramural
Fibroids

Pedunculated
Submucosal Fibroid

Pedunculated
Subserosal Fibroid

Subserosal
Fibroid

Submucosal
Fibroid

Fibroid Uterus

How Are Uterine Fibroids Discovered?

Uterine fibroids are usually discovered during a routine pelvic examination. During the examination, the doctor is able to feel an enlarged uterus or a pelvic mass. If a doctor thinks that fibroids are present and the uterus has grown to at least the size of a twelve-week pregnancy, he will sometimes immediately recommend a hysterectomy without any further tests.

Here's one, very emphatic, piece of sisterly advice: INSIST ON FURTHER TESTS! Do not, let me repeat, do **NOT** go from a simple physical examination directly to the surgical suite for a hysterectomy. In at least one major hospital review of hysterectomies where the uterus was removed purely because of the diagnosis of uterine fibroids, up to **9 percent** of the uteri were completely normal. No fibroids. No disease whatsoever. **Nine percent**. Apparently, the diagnosis of uterine fibroids by manual examination of the uterus is not without its problems.

To confirm the diagnosis of uterine fibroids, your doctor should request some form of imaging examination. An ultrasound, magnetic resonance imaging (MRI), hysterosonogram, hysteroscopy, or laparoscopy is usually scheduled. Imaging tests can tell your doctor approximately how big your uterus is, how many fibroids you have, their size, and their location. In addition, endometrial polyps or hyperplasia (an abnormal development of cells) can be visualized as well as ovarian cysts, masses, and endometriosis. Sometimes imaging can also reveal specific characteristics of fibroids such as whether or not they are degenerating or dying. With an MRI, the presence of adenomyosis (endometrial tissue invasion of the myometrium) can also be determined.

Ultrasound

A pelvic ultrasound is the most common type of imaging test done, primarily because it is the least expensive option. In most cases, two different types of ultrasound are done: transabdominal and transvaginal. Prior to a transabdominal ultrasound, you are requested to drink what seems like an impossible quantity of water, particularly when you have fibroids already taking up a lot of abdominal space and pressing against your bladder. There just doesn't seem as if there's any room left for drinking a great deal of water and the pressure to urinate can increase significantly. Don't be tempted to relieve your bladder—the water you've consumed is quite necessary for this test.

Once you've consumed an adequate quantity of water, a technician directs you to a testing room and instructs you to put on a hospital gown.

Then, while you're lying down on a table, the technician squirts a special type of jelly on your abdomen. A probe (transducer) is moved over your abdomen to get a reading. High-frequency waves bouncing off your inner organs (and all that water you just drank) create pictures.

The transvaginal portion of the ultrasound is done next and involves inserting a probe into your vagina. There is good news, however. You get to empty your bladder before this portion of the ultrasound is done! With this test, you have the option of placing the probe into your vagina by yourself. Most technicians will ask whether or not you would prefer this option, as some women do feel more comfortable inserting it themselves. However, the technician still needs to control the probe and move it around within the vagina to get the necessary images.

Hysterosonogram

When a transvaginal ultrasound is done, it is also possible to inject a small amount of water into the uterine cavity so that the lining of the uterus is more clearly defined. This procedure is called a hysterosonogram and is useful in differentiating between an endometrial polyp and a submucosal fibroid.

Magnetic Resonance Imaging (MRI)

Magnetic Resonance Imaging (MRI) is currently the most accurate way to diagnose uterine fibroids. In addition to location, size, and quantity of fibroids, it can fairly accurately tell your doctor the condition of your fibroids. MRI is also much better than ultrasound for telling the difference between a subserosal fibroid and some other form of mass in your uterus. Some doctors will bypass the ultrasound entirely and go straight to an MRI to get better images of your uterus. It is, however, more expensive and some insurance providers may protest or deny coverage when it is used. If you are concerned about this possibility, it may be wise to check with your insurer before undergoing an MRI.

While you don't have to drink a ton of water to have an MRI test, you do have to lie still on a flat "bed" of sorts that moves through a tunnel-like piece of equipment. It can be claustrophobic and noisy and if you happen to be overweight you may not even fit through the opening of this machine. Newer MRI equipment is "open," doesn't go through a tunnel, and can handle larger-sized individuals. Since MRI does use magnetic sources of energy to acquire an image, anyone who has metal implants of any kind may want to discuss the use of alternative imaging techniques for the diagnosis of her uterine fibroids.

Hysteroscopy

Hysteroscopy uses a slender instrument (the hysteroscope) to help the doctor see inside the uterus. It is inserted through the vagina and cervix and allows the doctor to see any fibroids located inside the uterine cavity. At the same time, he can take a look at your uterine lining and see whether any polyps are present. Hysteroscopy can occur in the doctor's office without anesthesia or on an outpatient basis at a hospital or clinic under general or regional anesthesia. If you've been experiencing excessive bleeding, your doctor might also perform a dilation and currettage (D&C) during the hysteroscopy to scrape out some of the uterine lining. Any necessary biopsies of the endometrial lining or polyps can also be taken during hysteroscopy.

Laparoscopy

Laparoscopy uses a slender instrument (the laparoscope) to help the doctor see inside the abdomen. The laparoscope is inserted through a small cut just below or through the navel. The doctor can see fibroids on the outside of the uterus as well as those that distort the shape of the body of the uterus. In addition, the fallopian tubes, ovaries, and surrounding pelvic region can all be visualized.

Laparoscopy is considered an outpatient surgical procedure and is done under regional or general anesthesia. Because of this, it is rarely used in the diagnosis of uterine fibroids. If a woman is experiencing a tremendous amount of pain that may be indicative of endometriosis, laparoscopy is used to establish a definitive diagnosis. This can be important because treatment options available to you for your uterine fibroids are impacted by the presence of endometriosis.

Can Uterine Fibroids Become Cancerous?

Here's the short answer. No. It doesn't happen. The long answer is that researchers and clinicians disagree on whether or not uterine fibroids actually can *become* cancerous—but it has never been *proven* to be the case. Uterine fibroids (leioyomyomas) and cancerous tumors of the uterus (leiomyosarcomas) do seem to be two entirely different beasts. They develop differently. They have different cellular structures. They even seem to be derived from different abnormal chromosomes.

So how do doctors even tell them apart? Well, generally speaking, they can't until they are removed and sent to the lab for analysis. That's definitely part of the problem with diagnosing cancerous tumors of the uterus. We do know, however, that leiomyosarcoma is most common in postmenopausal women in their fifties and sixties and occur around **1 percent** of the time (1 in 100) for that age bracket and older. Sudden growths of a tumor or abnormal bleeding in a postmenopausal woman are two signs of the potential presence of a cancerous tumor.

On the other hand, for premenopausal women the risk of those tumors being cancerous and not simply benign uterine fibroids is only around **.1 percent** (1 in 1,000). Sudden tumor growth and/or excessive bleeding is **not,** necessarily, a sign of leiomyosarcoma at all but simply an indicator of hormonal imbalance and pressure on the uterine lining due to the presence of the fibroids.

But what about those "rapidly growing" fibroids we hear so much about—you know, the ones that will get you an immediate recommendation for a hysterectomy from your gynecologist? As it turns out, in 320 cases where "rapidly growing fibroids" were actually diagnosed and hysterectomies were performed, there was only a **.25 percent** incidence of malignancy. A **.25 percent** incidence of cancer would roughly represent only **5** women out of **2,000** who were actually *diagnosed with rapidly growing fibroids* who would benefit from the life-saving measure of removing their uterus. The other 1,995 or **99.75 percent** may well represent an awful lot of unnecessary surgery.

With such a small number of cancerous tumors growing in women's bodies, it's hard for researchers to nail this one down and say for certain whether or not uterine fibroids can *become* cancerous. Most researchers now believe that uterine fibroids and cancerous tumors are two different types of tumors that grow independently of each other. The real answer, however, is simply unknown and the subject is still out for debate and in need of more definitive research.

Fibroids and Infertility

Fibroids can be a serious problem for women who desire pregnancy. They can completely prevent a successful pregnancy from occurring by interfering in the following ways:

- Submucosal fibroids take up space in the endometrium and can prevent a fertilized egg from implanting.
- Fibroids located near the fallopian tubes can obstruct the passageway, making it impossible for sperm to go up and eggs to come down.
- Fibroids compete for the blood supply of the uterus and often win out over any developing fetus.
- Cervical fibroids distort the cervix and possibly affect the cervical mucus, interfering with the sperm.

Many women have been known to carry a child full term even when fibroids were present. I did. Twice. Regardless, the amount of estrogen generated during a pregnancy can cause the fibroids to grow right along with the developing fetus and can make the pregnancy difficult, if not impossible, for many women.

Although there isn't any clinical research that shows removing fibroids increase your changes of becoming pregnant and carrying a child to full term, it certainly makes sense that it *might* help. **All other possible reasons for infertility should be ruled out first, however, particularly if your fibroids aren't causing you any other noticeable symptoms.**

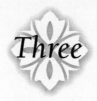

Three

The Choices

Currently, there isn't a *cure* for the disease of uterine fibroids. As I indicated in chapter 1, *Why Me?* doctors don't really know *why* fibroids become symptomatic in the first place and they certainly haven't progressed to the point of coming up with a cure yet either.

Since over 25 percent of all women are faced with symptomatic uterine fibroids at some point in their lifetime and doctors have known and written about uterine fibroids for over 150 years, one might think that medical science had figured this one out by now. It hasn't. Although researchers are working on this issue, currently no such cure exists.

The Choices for treatment currently fall into three primary categories:

1. **Ignore the Fibroids** (and any symptoms you may be experiencing).
2. **Treat the Symptoms** that are the result of symptomatic fibroids. With a bit of trial-and-error effort, symptoms that are the result of uterine fibroids are often treatable. The most common symptoms of uterine fibroids are:
   - abnormal bleeding (menorrhagia)
   - anemia, fatigue (generally the result of abnormal bleeding)
   - chronic pelvic pain or pelvic pressure
   - urinary frequency
   - constipation
3. **Treat the Fibroids** using one of the following treatment options:
   - myomectomy (laparoscopy, hysteroscopy, laparotomy)

➤ uterine artery embolization
➤ myolysis / cryomyolysis
➤ hysterectomy
➤ clinical trials / research

Generally speaking, most gynecologists encourage ignoring the fibroids and treating whatever symptoms occur as much as possible up until the point where the fibroids and uterus reach a size equivalent to a twelve-week pregnancy. Then, provided the woman does not desire additional children, the American College of Obstetricians and Gynecologists recommends only one treatment option: hysterectomy. (For details on the **ACOG Uterine Fibroids and Hysterectomy Criteria,** see chapter 6, "Treat the Fibroids.") In addition, some gynecologists will offer a hysterectomy as a way to treat the symptoms, regardless of the size of the uterus and fibroids.

Every gynecologist is different, sees a different set of patients, and formulates opinions about all patients based on their own set of experiences with their own patients. In addition to their contact with patients, their medical school training and residency all work together to form the foundation for why, what, and how any given physician recommends specific courses of treatment to their patients. This can be very different from one doctor to the next.

What many doctors fail to understand, though, is just how much *their* input of information shapes the choices that women make. Based on their own training and experiences with patients, they readily formulate opinions about the choices women will make in treating their uterine fibroids—but then completely fail to understand that their very own input of information may have caused that choice to be made.

It's quite possible that many physicians do **not** present information impartially and it's also quite probable that they do not offer complete information on all the potential treatment choices. For example, many doctors won't offer a treatment choice that they themselves cannot or do not want to perform. Myomectomy is performed fewer than 40,000 times a year for the treatment of uterine fibroids—compared with an average of 270,000 hysterectomies performed for the same disease.

Performing a successful and safe myomectomy requires surgical skill along with the willingness to take the additional time necessary to perform the procedure. Laparoscopic and hysteroscopic myomectomy are procedures that require skill some physicians may not have acquired during medical school. In addition, limited training in performing procedures with the laparoscope and hysteroscope can also be a hindrance. As a result of these factors and more, many physicians hesitate to recommend myomectomy to their patients.

Avoiding a surgical switch to hysterectomy midway through a myomectomy is more probable when the physician doing the surgery frequently performs myomectomies and also, perhaps, holds a basic belief that the uterus serves a function beyond childbearing and is worth retaining unless cancer is present.

Over time, some physicians may come to believe that hysterectomy is actually the treatment of choice by women when it is much more likely that they, as physicians, played a tremendous role in that choice. Medical decisions are most often based on the information that is presented to a patient—information presented by the physician. What woman would choose myomectomy when a physician describes it in a way that makes hysterectomy seem far superior? And what is a woman to do when her trusted gynecologist of many years ONLY recommends hysterectomy and discounts all other treatment options?

Why have approximately 7.5 million women had their ovaries prophylactically removed (during the performance of a hysterectomy) in the United States over the past twenty years even when no ovarian disease was present? Because it was recommended by the physician. The vast majority of women do not walk into doctors' offices and ask for the removal of their ovaries along with the uterus. It just doesn't happen. Choosing oophorectomy is not like choosing french fries to go with a hamburger!

Did the women making the choice to have their ovaries removed as a preventive measure against ovarian cancer have all the necessary information presented to them in order to make an objective decision on this matter? With a less than 1.8 percent lifetime risk of even developing ovarian cancer, I must wonder. Why would nearly half a million women a year have their ovaries removed when they had only a 1.8 percent chance of acquiring ovarian cancer? What DID their physician tell them?

Influencing the Patient

Many doctors sincerely believe that they present impartial and completely unbiased information to their patients regarding treatment options for uterine fibroids. They also believe that they allow the patient to freely make her own choices regarding her care and treatment. There are, however, many examples in medical research that clearly show the strong impact of physician input on treatment decisions that are made by the patient.

A striking and controversial example of this occurred in Finland during the past twenty years. Dr. P. Kilkku, a gynecologist at the Turku University Central Hospital in Finland, conducted research on the impact of hysterectomy on urinary and sexual symptoms. As a result of that research, which concluded that subtotal hysterectomies provided greater results with urinary and sexual function over total hysterectomies, subtotal hysterectomies have become very popular the world over. Subsequent research by Dr. H. S. Virtenan from the very same institute, however, has prompted editorial commentary in medical journals such as the following:

"The real current debate, however, is whether subtotal hysterectomy confers any benefits over total hysterectomy. In a series of publications from 1983, Kilkku extolled the virtues of subtotal hysterectomy with respect to urinary and sexual function, such that in Finland, where Kilkku carried out his studies, 53% of abdominal hysterectomies from 1981 to 1986 were subtotal."

There is little doubt that Dr. Kilkku pointed out his own research findings to every patient he encountered, thus further influencing them to undergo a subtotal hysterectomy. But were his research and recommendation valid?

*"However, subsequent studies by Virtanen et al. from the **same institute** did **not** concur with Kilkku's findings and by 1991 the rate of subtotal hysterectomy had dropped to 13%."*

The number of subtotal hysterectomies performed dropped from 53 percent to 13 percent in only five short years—simply because of different physicians influencing patients during different time periods at the very same hospital. Both Dr. Kilkku and Dr. Virtanen conducted "research" that they believed to be valid in supporting their own recommendations to women for subtotal or total hysterectomy.

Depending upon which side of the fence gynecologists fall on with the issue of total versus subtotal hysterectomy, they will generally cite one of these studies to support their recommendation—rarely do they cite BOTH studies so that patients can read them both and decide for themselves. This kind of bias in reporting of published research to patients is outrageous—but practiced by many doctors.

The bottom line on this whole issue is simple. Whether doctors admit it or not, every single word that they say to their patients matters and has a driving influence on the decisions that are made. For many physicians this is truly a hard concept to grasp. Even harder yet is learning to temper and "frame" the information presented to patients appropriately and without bias.

But this is a two-way street. Patients **must** become more involved in learning about their own medical condition and take the time to ask questions. Lots of them. Seek out second opinions. Ask more questions. Learn as much as possible about the medical condition and treatment options *before* consenting to a specific treatment plan. Until this level of patient involvement occurs, it's impossible to say that physicians really know or can adequately predict what a patient with true knowledge of all available options will choose.

Information about treatment choices is presented in chapters 4, 5, and 6 and provides information about the three primary treatment choice categories:

- Ignore the fibroids.
- Treat the symptoms.
- Treat the fibroids.

With each of these treatment choice categories, details about the options currently available are presented. I hope that the information throughout the following chapters will provide you with additional treatment options to consider, help you to weigh the benefits and risks of each option, fill in any gaps of information that your physician may have left out, and, quite possibly, help you to better understand and potentially avoid making the ACOG-recommended decision to undergo hysterectomy for the treatment of your benign uterine fibroids and their accompanying symptoms.

A Few Words about Drugs, Devices, and the FDA

In the United States, the Food and Drug Administration (FDA) is responsible for overseeing the safety of consumers in the purchase and use of all foods, drugs, and medical devices.

There are many drugs and treatment devices currently on the market prescribed or used by physicians for the treatment of symptoms resulting from uterine fibroids or for the treatment of the uterine fibroids themselves. There are even more herbal remedies and creams that patients themselves have direct, over-the-counter access to purchasing in their desire to find relief from the multitude of symptoms that may be accompanying their uterine fibroids.

Herbal remedies, shark cartilage, and progesterone creams available for purchase over-the-counter are not chemical compounds that are government regulated. At this time, NONE of these remedies have had thorough studies completed that demonstrate their ability to alleviate symptoms of uterine fibroids, diminish the size of uterine fibroids, or eliminate uterine fibroids. Furthermore, because they are not government regulated they are not required to prove their efficacy and, as a result, you will not find a single over-the-counter product labeled specifically for the treatment of uterine fibroids or their accompanying symptoms. It is important to keep this in mind when reviewing the variety of treatment options available for uterine fibroid symptoms within the following chapters.

In addition to the non-government-regulated remedies available, there is a variety of additional drugs and devices that should also be approached with caution as you carefully weigh the benefits and risks of treatment options for your specific condition. Lupron, for instance, is a gonadotropin-releasing hormone often prescribed to shrink fibroids. Polyvinyl alcohol particles (PVA) are considered "devices" used to stop the blood flow to the fibroids and also shrink them. Needles or cryoprobes used in myolysis and cryomyolysis are also considered "devices," as are thermal ablation devices used in endometrial ablation. All these items fall under the guidelines requiring FDA oversight and regulation for consumer protection. But have any of these drugs or devices actually been approved by the FDA for the specific treatment of uterine fibroids?

It's a tricky question and one that will get you a wide variety of answers and explanations. Lupron, for example, has in fact been approved—for the treatment of prostate cancer in men. However, it didn't take long before gynecologists began using this drug for a wide variety of hormonally related conditions in women, including the shrinking of uterine fibroids. Was it approved? Yes. For the specific treatment of uterine fibroids? No. This is what is called an "off-label" use of a government-regulated product. Physicians regularly use a wide variety of drugs and devices in this manner and, sometimes, place the patient at risk in doing so. *Note: More recently, Lupron did receive approval for short-term use (no more than six months in the lifetime of a woman) for assistance in alleviating symptoms associated with endometriosis and also to induce temporary menopause so that excessive bleeding would subside and allow a woman's hematocrit* (red blood cell ratio) *to return to normal prior to surgery for uterine fibroids. It has NOT, however, been approved for "shrinking fibroids."*

Only YOU—not your physician—should ultimately decide which risks are worth taking for the treatment of your uterine fibroids. Since many different drugs and devices are used to treat both the symptoms and the fibroids (often *off-label*), it's certainly wise to work *with* your physician in discussing all the information and options available to you but, ultimately, it should be *your* decision. Consider the following:

- Before accepting medication your physician prescribes (including in-office injections), ask to see any product insert datasheets (PIDs) or patient brochures that have been created by the manufacturer that describe the FDA-approved use of the product, contraindications, and side effects. You can ask your physician for this information and you can also request a copy of the PID or brochure from your pharmacist before having your prescription filled.
- Before undergoing a procedure that involves the use of medical devices, find out if they've been approved for the particular procedure by, again, asking to see the product insert datasheet. Every device approved by the FDA that is sold to a physician comes with a PID or product brochure. If the device is going to be implanted in your body (as PVA is with uterine artery embolization), INSIST upon reviewing the information written and provided by the manufacturer with the physician.

Admittedly, product insert datasheets can sometimes be difficult to read. Don't be afraid to ask your physician or pharmacist a lot of questions. They should be willing and available to share the information contained in a product insert datasheet and clarify any items that you don't understand.

As the patient and a consumer, you have a right to read this information—but it is up to you to actually obtain copies. Make it a habit to ask—a common practice to request and receive product insert datasheets or patient brochures. Then read them!

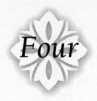

Four

Ignore the Fibroids

So. You have uterine fibroids and the first treatment option that comes spilling out of your doctor's mouth is *hysterectomy*. You either sit there in shock—you truly had no idea that that is what the doctor would say— or, you take your doctor very seriously and begin a discussion regarding the time frame to schedule the surgery.

Take a deep breath. Pause to clear your head as much as possible. Then, proceed to make that doctor work **hard** for that diagnosis and recommendation for hysterectomy. For a starter, have you had any of those diagnostic tests (such as ultrasound or magnetic resolution imaging) that I discussed in chapter 2, *Anatomy of a Fibroid,* which would give you more information about your fibroids? If you have abnormal bleeding, have you had an endometrial biopsy? If you're tired all the time and run-down, have you had blood tests to determine your hematocrit? If you have urinary incontinence or painful urination, has anyone bothered to check for an infection? Back up from that surgery and take your fibroid situation one step at a time.

Learn everything you can about your fibroids and available treatment options BEFORE you jump off the treatment choice cliff. Once you choose and undergo a hysterectomy, there is simply no turning back. Millions of women have jumped off that cliff blindly and many of them regret it to this day. Logging on to the Internet and doing a search on "hysterectomy" will bring you support groups where women express over and over again how much they wish they had taken more time to truly research and understand the potential consequences of this procedure. Many regret their decision to undergo hysterectomy but are trying to learn coping skills and share medical information in an effort to help one another through what is a difficult recovery time for them.

> The thought that is running through my mind, without fail, is "I wish I had never had this surgery." It is with me every minute of every day. I don't think I will ever be truly happy, healthy, or at peace with my body. It has truly ruined my life, and irrevocably changed the lives of my husband and children.
> —DeeDee

Still others simply wish they'd taken into consideration more information regarding keeping their cervix intact or the impact on their overall hormone levels with the removal of their ovaries. Surgical menopause can be extremely difficult on a woman, and balancing those missing hormones can be a time-consuming and troublesome feat.

Uterine fibroids are not generally life threatening and, as such, treatment choices are considered *elective* options. In other words, while it may seem like your doctor is telling you that you MUST have a hysterectomy to treat your fibroids, the reality is that you do not *have* to do anything about treating your uterine fibroids. A hysterectomy performed for the treatment of *benign* uterine fibroids is considered **elective** surgery that you, the patient, have *freely chosen to undergo.* The same statement can be made for every treatment choice available for uterine fibroids.

So ask questions. Learn more. Find out what kind of fibroids you have, how big they are, where they are located and what ALL your options may be to treat either your fibroids or simply the symptoms you may be experiencing (for example, excessive bleeding or urinary incontinence).

Don't accept a two-minute dog-and-pony show presenting maybe only one other *possible* treatment choice, where the doctor shows you a pretty graphic, points to pictures of female parts, but doesn't really give you enough details for you to truly comprehend the information just presented. The graphics are usually flip charts or handouts with little to no real content on them. Maybe the physician allows questions—maybe he/she cuts you off, politely and authoritatively of course. But, it sounds good. The pictures might even look good.

Snap Out of It!

Think: Advertising. Was the time the doctor just spend discussing your options shorter or longer than a ***60-second commercial?***

These presentations almost always end with the doctor completely discounting all other options and recommending proceeding with only the hysterectomy option. You might even get a comic book or videotape handed to you to take home and review as I did on multiple occasions. *(Pay close attention to who funded the printing of those materials! There are many, many people who have a vested financial interest in your decision regarding hysterectomy.)*

Don't just sit there and gloss over it all. Look that doctor square in the eye and ask the following question:

*"So, Doc: Tell me what will happen if I choose to **Ignore the Fibroids?**"*

I can't stress this enough. Get off that freight train bound for immediate hysterectomy territory and at least *try* to get a satisfactory answer to the above question before you do anything else. If your fibroids truly aren't causing you any problems, there isn't any reason at all for you to take any treatment action—especially not hysterectomy.

Let me repeat: Take a deep breath. Ask questions. Learn more. If you are experiencing troublesome symptoms, the doctor should be running diagnostic tests—not running you into surgery. Find out **what kind of fibroids you have, how big they are, where they are located,** and **what ALL your options are for simply treating the symptoms you may be experiencing OR the fibroids.** But whatever you do, do **not** let your doctor get away with a simple dog-and-pony show in an attempt to convince you to undergo surgery.

The Doctor Answers

Okay. So you asked the questions. Maybe you got direct answers and maybe you didn't. Maybe you got the following statement thrown in for good measure:

"Well, the fibroids seem to be growing rapidly and there's always the possibility that the fibroids are cancerous or could become cancerous."

Ding ding ding ding ding. Did a warning bell just go off in your head? It should have. We talked about this in chapter 2, *Anatomy of a Fibroid.* The chances are slim to none that your fibroids are cancerous. Remember, less than **1 percent** of all fibroids are malignant. Is it possible? Yes. Have any of your symptoms forbode cancer? Has the doctor run any tests that have made him believe that the presence of cancer is real? Or, was this simply one of the first things the doctor chose to tell you, possibly in an attempt to convince you to have a hysterectomy? Listen carefully to how your physician phrases the potential for cancer with your uterine fibroids. Statements like ". . . there's always the possibility . . ." or ". . . cancer cannot be ruled out . . ." are not, necessarily, false statements. They are, however, misleading statements that do not truly give you the opportunity to assess the actual presence or risk of cancer with your uterine fibroids.

Rapidly Growing Fibroids

A majority of women presenting with fibroids are told they have "rapidly growing fibroids," but no one really knows what they are or what is meant by the term. Apparently all that rapid growing spells trouble—potential cancer—immediate need for a hysterectomy.

A LOT of women have heard this story. A LOT of women are frightened by these words.

Realistic statistics on true incidence of cancerous fibroids (less than 1 percent) would place the status of this story into the **urban legend from the gynecological underworld** category.

I've corresponded and spoken with thousands of women who've heard the "rapidly growing fibroids" story from their gynecologist or general practitioner. Many of them underwent hysterectomy within two weeks of hearing this "story."

Others chose to get a second opinion. NONE of them presented with a malignant fibroid.

So what is, exactly, the definition of a rapidly growing fibroid?

Any uterus increasing in gestational size of six weeks or more during the course of an entire year could be considered to have a rapidly growing fibroid tumor. This is dependent upon size verification with *ultrasound*

MRI and then, one year later, a second check—again with *ultrasound* or *MRI*—to determine the growth during the course of the year.

Recent research, however, has shown that even when a fibroid is diagnosed as rapidly growing, it is cancerous less than 3 in 1,000 cases. *Only* **.25 percent** *of rapidly growing fibroids are truly cancerous!*

Obviously, no one should take the risk of cancer lightly. However, you might want to think seriously about the low risk factors presented in the preceding paragraph and discuss with your physician in greater depth the probability of whether or not *the diagnosis really* **is** *cancer* before you choose a surgical option that may be entirely unnecessary and change the quality of your life forever.

Okay. Let's put our logical thinking caps on. For every answer your doctor gives you, ask these questions:

- *"What's the likelihood of that happening?"*
- *"Can you tell me what the current statistics from the National Cancer Institute are regarding my actual risks for cancer?"*
- *"What's the worst thing that could happen to me if that did actually occur?"*
- *"What preventive measures, other than hysterectomy, can I take that would reduce the chances of that actually occurring?"*
- *"What tests can I undergo to rule out cancer prior to making a treatment decision?"*
- *"If cancer is present, would a hysterectomy improve my quality of life or lengthen it at all? Does the type of cancer present make a difference in your answer to this question or make a difference in the type of hysterectomy that should be performed? How so?*

Weigh each answer your doctor gives you very carefully. Know what the answer means, specifically, to you. Each person must weigh the risks of ignoring the fibroids against her own specific circumstances of physical condition, age, and beliefs and attitudes regarding her uterus and long-term health situation. Maybe you **are** in need of a hysterectomy. But, then again, maybe you **aren't.** Maybe, just maybe, there is another solution entirely that will allow you to retain your uterus and avoid the long list of potential complications from hysterectomy that currently plague a great many women who went forward with surgery before considering alternatives.

But I Can't Ignore the Fibroids

Do any of the following questions apply to your situation that make it impossible for you to *ignore the fibroids?*

- Are you experiencing unbearable symptoms from your fibroids?
- Is the pain more than you can tolerate another day longer?
- Is your bleeding so far out of control that you **hemorrhage** more than eight days out of every month and your periods barely stop before they begin again?
- Are you feeling weak and fatigued—possibly due to anemia brought on by excessive bleeding?
- How close in age are you to menopause and can you tolerate your current symptoms until your body goes through menopause?
- Are your fibroids becoming so large that they protrude and are uncomfortable?
- Is *ignoring the fibroids* simply not an option for you?

Ask yourself all these questions and more. Then, if you find that you simply can't *ignore the fibroids,* review all your options in the following two chapters very carefully. Learn as much as you can about your condition and work closely with a physician you truly trust. It's still possible that you have options other than hysterectomy. Find out. Ask the questions.

Okay. I've Weighed the Risks.
I'll Ignore the Fibroids.

If you do choose to *ignore the fibroids,* and postpone any kind of treatment for the time being, please stop and consider that perhaps something in your body is not quite right. Something is amiss. Your hormones are definitely sending you a signal that something is out of balance. You should at least attempt to read the message and discuss what it may mean with your physician. Maybe it means nothing and there isn't any reason to do anything. But then again, maybe it does mean something. Along with the help of a trusted physician, you can try to find out just what that something is and, perhaps, make changes that *might* alter the course of continued growth of your fibroids. It's important to work *with* your doctor on this medical condition and to not simply walk away from the situation—pretending as though it doesn't exist. If you've been diagnosed with uterine fibroids, it's incredibly important that you continue to seek care and monitor your condition so that, should your fibroids become unbearably symptomatic, you and your doctor will have a plan of action for treatment—preferably, one that allows you to retain your uterus and avoid an "emergency" hysterectomy.

Five

Treat the Symptoms

This chapter identifies many of the symptoms that can accompany uterine fibroids. In addition, it covers a variety of treatment options currently available that are used by patients and their physicians in an attempt to treat the physical symptoms often caused by uterine fibroids. None are absolute cures in treating the symptoms as they do not, let me repeat, **do not** treat the fibroids themselves. There is absolutely no documented evidence that any of these treatments will provide a "cure" for your uterine fibroids. Nonetheless, depending on the individual, any one of these treatment methods may bring some relief from the *symptoms* you may be experiencing as a result of your fibroids. In a sense, when symptoms are resolved, most patients feel "cured" and find no need to take additional action when it comes to their uterine fibroids.

Menorrhagia—Hemorrhagia— Abnormal Uterine Bleeding

One of the few things researchers do know about fibroids is that progesterone and estrogen seem to play a role in their development. It is not clear precisely what that role is, but simply that it is somehow related. With changes in hormonal levels, a wide variety of *symptoms* may occur, in addition to fibroids themselves.

Abnormal bleeding from the uterus is a very real possibility when hormonal imbalances occur, and an extremely bothersome symptom. Remember back in chapter 2, *Anatomy of a Fibroid,* when you read about the role of luteinizing hormones (LH) in your menstrual cycle? Well, normally your LH set off the release of eggs (ovulation) and progesterone levels in the ovaries go up. The progesterone level continually rises until about a week before the end of the menstrual cycle and then it decreases. When your progesterone level decreases, it is basically telling your body to get rid of the uterine lining that has built up for that month. However, if your luteinizing hormones stop functioning properly and ovulation doesn't occur, the progesterone level doesn't rise and can't send a signal telling your body to get rid of the uterine lining. At the same time, estrogen stimulates the endometrium to keep right on growing. Eventually, overdeveloped endometrial tissue starts to fall apart and this can lead to abnormal bleeding. Spotting, heavy menstrual bleeding, passing blood clots, delayed periods, or even bleeding throughout the entire month are all typical ways abnormal bleeding presents itself. In addition, bleeding is often aggravated and intensified by any fibroids that develop.

Normal menstrual periods generally last four to five days, but women with hormonal imbalances and fibroids often have periods lasting longer than seven days. Actually, that's putting it mildly. The real truth is that fibroids can cause bleeding to run wild. Some women end up changing sanitary pads every hour and doubling up with super-plus tampons. Even with double protection, a woman might STILL find herself flooding massively the minute she tries to walk out the door.

Abnormal bleeding can happen with any of the different types of uterine fibroids. Pure pelvic pressure from the size of the growing fibroid uterus alone can bring on massive bleeding—the larger the fibroid uterus, the more horrific it can become. Submucosal fibroids are by far the worst, because of their location on the endometrium. They create constant pressure against the uterine lining that builds with each menstrual cycle. Submucosal fibroids are often accompanied by continual, heavy bleeding.

Although rarely causing life-threatening conditions, abnormal blood loss from fibroids can be very dangerous. Even so, many women choose to simply *"ignore"* this heavy bleeding and avoid medical intervention. Some choose to take nonsteroidal anti-inflammatory drugs (NSAIDs)— like Ibuprofen™—to try to control the bleeding and accompanying menstrual pain. Unfortunately, NSAIDs aren't really very effective, and continued excessive bleeding typically leads to fatigue and anemia. In extreme cases and if ignored too long, excessive bleeding can become life threatening.

In addition to fibroids, abnormal bleeding can also be the result of a number of other benign conditions of the uterus, including any of the following:

➤ Von Willebrand's disease
➤ hypothyroidism
➤ liver disease
➤ chronic endometritis (a uterine infection)
➤ cervical polyps
➤ endometrial polyps
➤ adenomyosis

On the other hand, there is always the possibility that abnormal bleeding is an early warning sign that a precancerous condition could be developing. The following are all extremely serious conditions of the uterus that can also cause abnormal bleeding:

➤ vaginal cancer
➤ cervical dysplasia (precancerous stage of cervical cancer)
➤ cervical cancer
➤ endometrial hyperplasia (precancerous stage of uterine cancer)
➤ uterine cancer

If you are experiencing abnormal bleeding, I can't encourage you enough to undergo a thorough physical exam and evaluation by a physician that includes a manual *pelvic examination,* a *Pap smear,* and an *endometrial biopsy.* Do not wait. Do not put it off. Make the appointment for an exam today and ask about these tests. Your life could depend on it.

During the pelvic exam, your doctor will feel the shape of your uterus and this is, typically, when fibroids are first discovered if they are present. Women who conscientiously undergo annual exams are typically quite surprised to learn about the presence of fibroids in their body. Symptoms do not accompany most fibroids in their early development stages. Therefore, suddenly hearing the news that fibroid tumors are growing in your uterus can be quite a shock. Even so, it's much better to determine their presence in the early stages of development than to ignore them entirely until symptoms are completely out of control and your abdomen is terribly distended from their growth. Learning about your fibroids at an early stage can give you ample opportunity to learn more about them and prepare yourself for potential symptoms and possible treatments.

A Pap smear is generally performed annually along with a pelvic examination. This ritual of health care is important to your overall well-being and allows your physician to catch any early warning signs of precancerous conditions. A Pap smear checks for changes in your cervix and is used to detect dysplasia, the precancerous stage of cervical cancer. This diagnostic test involves scraping cells from your cervix and sending them to a lab for analysis. A Pap smear is not painful (for the majority of women) and takes only a few minutes to perform.

While the word *biopsy* does sound a bit frightening, an endometrial biopsy is actually a fairly simple and quick extraction of tissue from the endometrial lining. It's performed in an examining room at your doctor's office. While some women experience little to no pain during this test, others have reported significant cramping. The presence of submucosal fibroids may complicate things and could present additional pain as well. If the potential pain or cramping from this procedure concerns you, it may be a good idea to discuss with your physician whether or not you should take pain medications prior to undergoing the procedure.

Instead of an endometrial biopsy, your doctor may suggest that a dilation and currettage (D&C) be performed to eliminate any excessive lining that has built up in the endometrium as well as get a tissue sample to send to the lab for analysis. This procedure is usually performed on an outpatient basis under general anesthesia. A D&C allows for the lining to be scraped away and gives you some temporary relief from the excessive bleeding. But it *is* temporary. Hormonal imbalances causing the endometrial lining to build up in the first place are certainly not treated with a D&C and, over time if left untreated, the lining is sure to build up again. For this reason, many doctors prescribe progestin in an attempt to regulate the progesterone in your body and to, hopefully, prevent another episode of excessive cell growth in the endometrium.

Changing Your Diet

For many years now there has been speculation that becoming a vegetarian may have an impact on the bleeding that occurs as a result of uterine fibroids. In fact, many women have indeed reported success at controlling their bleeding through the simple elimination of meat from their daily diet.

> *"I changed my diet (excluded red meat and dairy) and started an exercise program. I also take vitamins and a calcium supplement. I have not had any problems with my fibroids in quite some time. My periods have returned to three days a month with only moderate flow. The bleeding has been under control for almost a year now."*
> —Jan

In 1999, new research from Italy was published in *Obstetrics & Gynecology* that finally showed an association between consumption of specific dietary items and uterine fibroids.

The researchers in Italy set out to analyze the relationship between diet and the risk of uterine fibroids. They collected data for eleven years from over two thousand women. The consumption of the following food items was determined to have a high association with uterine fibroids:

➤ beef
➤ red meat (other than beef)
➤ ham

An additional PROTECTIVE association was made with the consumption of the following food items:

➤ green vegetables
➤ fruit
➤ fish

The most important item with the highest protective association was green vegetables—the number one food group that many of us struggle to consume enough of on a daily basis!

Although the consumption of these few food items listed above was either positively or negatively associated with uterine fibroids, it's important to point out that researchers were **not** able to determine an increased risk of fibroids associated with the consumption of any of the following items:

> milk
> liver
> carrots
> eggs
> whole-grain foods
> butter
> margarine
> oil
> coffee
> tea
> alcohol

It is equally important to point out that researchers were not studying whether or not eating certain foods would alter the *symptoms* women experience with uterine fibroids, such as abnormal bleeding. They were only looking for dietary associations that could be matched with the presence or absence of uterine fibroids. Therefore, it is not known whether or not altering your diet after uterine fibroids are diagnosed would, in fact, have an impact on abnormal bleeding or fibroid growth. Even so, modifying your diet by reducing the amount of beef, other red

"After being diagnosed with fibroids, I changed to a vegan diet (no meat and no dairy products), with the exception of fish (particularly salmon and tuna). I try to eat more whole foods concentrating on grains and vegetables. I can't really say if the change in diet has made a difference in halting the growth of my fibroids. We'll see as time goes on, but I did lose about five pounds and feel much better."

—Janet

meat, and ham you eat and increasing your vegetable, fruit, and fish in-take would represent a more balanced and healthier diet. Although re-search doesn't exist that proves its impact on symptoms, many women have indicated they received some relief from their symptoms through a change in diet.

Castor Oil Packs

Castor oil packs are a rather intriguing treatment option that involves taking a flannel cloth, soaking it in castor oil and applying it to the ab-domen. Many women's health books discussing treatments for the symp-toms of uterine fibroids suggest the use of castor oil packs. This has always perplexed me somewhat as there never seems to be a reasonable explanation that accompanies this "remedy" and there are never any ref-erences indicating where in the world this suggestion originated.

There has been no scientific research to date that studies the impact of castor oil packs on uterine fibroids or their symptoms, such as bleeding. However, castor oil packs have been used for thousands of years throughout the world for a wide variety of ailments. Aztecs used them for treatment of skin lesions and hemorrhoids, Persians used them for epilepsy, the Greek Dioscorides used them for the reduction of tumors, and the Egyptians used them for eye irritation. More recently, there has been research identifying castor oil packs applied abdominally as an anti-toxin that has an impact on the lymphatic delivery system.

In 1999, a paper entitled "Immunomodulation Through Castor Oil Packs," written by Harvey Grady, was published in the *Journal of Naturo-pathic Medicine*. This paper details the results of a double-blind study done on thirty-six healthy subjects before and after applying castor oil packs abdominally for two hours daily while having them rest in bed.

As medical studies go, this one was very small and carried out for the sole purpose of attempting to identify whether this topical treatment had any impact on the lymphatic delivery system or not. The results? With a minimal two-hour therapy period, this study found that castor oil packs produced a "significant" temporary increase in the number of T-11 cells that increased over a seven hour period following treatment and then re-turned to normal levels within 24 hours later.

"The T-11 cell increase represents a general boost in the body's specific de-

fense status. Lymphocytes actively defend the health of the body by forming an-
tibodies against pathogens and their toxins. T-cell lymphocytes originate from
bone marrow and the thymus gland as small lymphocytes that identify and kill
viruses, fungi, bacteria, and cancer cells. T-11 cell lymphocytes supply a fun-
damental antibody capability to keep the specific defense system strong."

In the Discussion section of the paper, the author suggested two possible theories for why the immune system is affected by topical treatment
with castor oil:

1. T-lymphocytes (which exist throughout the skin) in the epidermis
   and upper dermis layers communicate with and influence the activity
   of the general immune system.
2. Prostaglandins activity is stimulated. Prostaglandins play a key role in
   regulating *cell division* in the body and are involved in your body's immune response.

While these are interesting theories, further investigation is necessary
before any conclusions can be drawn in terms of whether or not castor oil
packs have any impact on uterine fibroids whatsoever. There simply isn't
enough information that might identify how or why castor oil packs may
or may not work on one's immune system or cell division (such as that
which occurs when fibroids are growing) to draw any medical conclusions about use of this treatment.

While naturopaths often recommend castor oil packs for uterine fibroids, they are equally quick to say that simply lying down for two
hours a day with a warm pack on the abdomen (with or without castor
oil) may provide the same benefit. There is simply insufficient science behind this age-old treatment to give us any real answers as to purported
benefits. Even so, many women are dedicated to seeking alternative
treatment options for their symptoms and are willing to try this naturopathic treatment.

If you do choose to try castor oil pack treatment, the following are tips
on how it should be applied:

1. Soak a flannel cloth thoroughly in castor oil (it should be soaked but
   not dripping).
2. Lying down, place the castor oil pack on your abdomen.

"I have read that using castor oil packs can shrink fibroids, but I haven't read any studies that prove this. I know that lack of research is an issue with alternative treatments. But I'll try just about anything that I don't think will hurt me and am trying castor oil packs now. I know there aren't any good studies that show they stop bleeding or shrink fibroids. That doesn't mean it won't work."
—Patty

3. Cover with plastic wrap and then a towel.
4. Keep in place for a minimum of 1 hour.

Some women apply this pack at night and sleep with it on. Since this can be a rather sticky and greasy treatment option, you may want to take precautions against getting the oil-soaked cloth on your clothing or bedding. Cleaning the skin afterwards can be done with a mixture of baking soda and water (two teaspoons of baking soda to a quart of water).

Because this treatment must be used every day of the week (even though it has not been proven that it has an impact on *bleeding* or the *growth* or *shrinkage* of the fibroids), my number one question with this treatment is: How many days in total should this be done? For as long as you have symptoms? For as long as the abnormal bleeding or fibroids are present? Forever? Using castor oil packs is a messy, time-consuming treatment that is difficult for most patients to continue for very long. Patient "compliance" with this daily treatment regimen is a HUGE issue and may be the reason why we don't know more than we do about its true impact on the immune system over long periods of use.

There are two primary benefits that some women seem to derive from this treatment:

1. stress relief (perhaps from lying down for an hour each day)
2. reduction in premenstrual syndrome symptoms

Neither of these benefits has anything to do with fibroid shrinkage or reduction in bleeding symptoms. In my own experience with castor oil packs, this remedy definitely didn't alter the growth of my fibroids or reduce the bleeding. I can say, however, that it did give me a very nice "quiet time" each day. This, in turn, helped to lower my stress level. That benefit alone may be a good enough reason to give this remedy a try.

Natural Remedies

Natural remedies for abnormal bleeding include everything from nutritional supplements (vitamins A, B-complex, C, K, and bioflavonoids) to botanical herbs (chaste tree, ginger, cranesbill, shepherd's purse, ragwort, blue cohosh, false unicorn) and natural progesterone. Self-treatment with natural remedies, particularly nutritional supplements and botannical herbs, without the advice and guidance of a naturopathic physician is not recommended. Combinations of herbs along with the correct dosing can be critical and, if done improperly, may be toxic. While it may be tempting to simply experiment with the wide variety of vitamin supplements and herbs that are available in the marketplace, most women who do so typically express a lack of understanding of what they are taking, its impact on the menstrual cycle, and, in the end, are frustrated and dissatisfied with the results. You probably wouldn't dream of mixing and matching prescription drugs at random in an effort to self-treat a medical condition; it doesn't make sense to mix and match vitamins and herbs without proper guidance either.

To locate a naturopathic physician near you, contact the American Association of Naturopathic Physicians:

American Association of Naturopathic Physicians (AANP)
8201 Greensboro Drive, Suite 300
McLean, Virginia 22102
703-610-9037
http://www.naturopathic.org

Only a couple of the most popular natural remedies for bleeding disorder are identified in this section. To learn more, an excellent resource and learning tool is the *Women's Encyclopedia of Natural Medicine: Alternative Therapies and Integrative Medicine,* by Dr. Tori Hudson. To date, this is the most comprehensive women's health book written that details naturopathic and botanical medicine specifically for women.

The most commonly used herbal remedy for bleeding is chaste tree, commonly known as and purchased as Vitex in the United States. This herbal remedy product is derived from the berries of the chaste tree that grows in the Mediterranean countries and Central Asia. Chaste tree is a remedy that was traditionally used for many different conditions related to the reproductive system of women—including the control of hemorrhaging after childbirth. It doesn't contain any hormones. It works on the pituitary gland to affect the production of luteinizing hormones (LH). You might recall from chapter 2, *Anatomy of a Fibroid,* that LH hormones are responsible for stimulating the production of progesterone.

Chaste tree is NOT a fast-acting remedy and may take four to six months to show any effects. If you become pregnant while taking chaste tree, you should immediately discontinue its use.

Another natural remedy is False Unicorn. This plant is native to Mississippi and grows throughout the southern region of the United States. Although chaste tree is most often taken alone, this remedy is generally taken *with* chaste tree and not by itself—which makes it difficult to determine its true medicinal benefit and how it works to reduce bleeding symptoms. Even so, the root of this plant has been used by Native Americans for many years for a wide variety of reproductive health conditions and is considered to have a sedative effect on the uterus, thereby reducing uterine contractions and cramping. Historically, women with a history of miscarriage were encouraged to use False Unicorn before, during, and after pregnancy.

Natural progesterone is made from extracts of Mexican wild yam or soybeans and is a chemical duplication of the progesterone produced by your own body. The most popular form of natural progesterone is a skin cream, but it is also available as an injection, sublingual tablet (a tablet that dissolves under the tongue), rectal or vaginal suppository, and oral capsule or tablet. Natural progesterone cream products should contain at least 400 mg of progesterone per ounce in order to be effective. One-fourth to one-half a teaspoon should be applied two to three times per day for twenty-one days and then discontinued for the week during your period. Progesterone cream is typically packaged with enough cream in a tube or jar to last one month, and some manufacturers do include dosing instruments to help guide you in determining the appropriate application amount of cream.

Oral Contraceptives/Progestin

The majority of abnormal bleeding in women is caused by hormonal ups and downs that create an imbalance of estrogen and progesterone. Hormones, such as birth control pills, progestin (synthetic progesterone), and progesterone, or thyroid medication may be prescribed to help regulate your periods and, quite possibly, help to get your abnormal bleeding under control.

Hormonal treatments may take a few months to actually work, but are an extremely simple way to treat abnormal bleeding and should always be an initial option to consider. Hormonal regulation of the menstrual cycle doesn't always work to stop abnormal bleeding—but when it does, no other treatment is generally needed.

Of course, you're probably wondering whether or not the hormones in these drug therapies are just going to feed your fibroids and make them even bigger and, ultimately, make your symptoms worse. Or, you might be wondering whether progestin, progesterone, or estrogen therapies can be used to actually cure your fibroids. After all, there is so much we simply

Bleeding, Hormone Therapy, and the Postmenopausal Woman

While research has shown that hormonal therapy doesn't seem to contribute to the growth of uterine fibroids, there does seem to be an exception to this statement. Normally, when a woman goes through menopause, her production of estrogen shuts down and her fibroids shrink and her symptoms dissipate. Yahoo! Unfortunately, many postmenopausal women with fibroids then begin taking hormone replacement therapy (HRT). I write the word unfortunately *for a reason. Several studies have now shown that abnormal bleeding in postmenopausal women can occur when fibroids resume growing with the introduction of HRT into a woman's system.*

My question: Why does hormonal therapy have an impact on fibroid growth postmenopausally but not before then, according to the current set of studies? Research. We need more research! There doesn't seem to be a solid answer to this question.

don't know about what triggers the growth of fibroids in the first place, but it does seem to be hormonally related, doesn't it? Isn't it possible that contraceptives could be a contributing factor actually causing the growth of uterine fibroids or, on the other hand, a potential remedy for regulating hormones and fixing the fibroid problem?

Well, researchers have considered these possibilities. Current studies show that oral contraceptives do not seem to be a contributing factor to the presence of symptomatic fibroids; nor do they seem to contribute to fibroid growth. In reality, fibroids were found in women long before oral contraceptives were invented or mass-produced for distribution.

In addition, contraceptives do not work as a "cure" for fibroids. Introducing hormones into your system to regulate your menstrual cycle to possibly gain control over abnormal bleeding is one thing, but hormones won't "cure" your uterine fibroids. So, what's the bottom line on this issue? More research is needed. The current "answers" we have are confusing and inconclusive and sometimes even contradictory.

Endometrial Ablation / Cryoablation

Through hysteroscopy, the endometrial lining can be completely destroyed with a variety of "ablation" techniques. Ablation involves the removal of tissue through cauterizing it or lasering. Cryoablation involves a freezing technique and represents only one of many new methods that are being developed in an effort to make endometrial ablation a more effective treatment for abnormal bleeding. Ablation typically controls bleeding 70 to 90 percent of the time, but long-term side effects are not

Cancer and Endometrial Ablation

The number one warning sign of uterine cancer is abnormal bleeding. Because endometrial ablation removes the uterine lining and stops all bleeding in the majority of women, there is some concern that endometrial cancer could go undetected in a woman who has undergone this procedure. It has not, however, proven to be the case thus far. It is, nonetheless, extremely important to discuss this possibility with your physician and closely monitor your health with annual visits and appropriate tests should you choose this procedure.

known. Submucosal fibroids must be removed prior to endometrial ablation through hysteroscopic myomectomy.

You might think that following this procedure a woman would no longer have bleeding from a monthly menstrual period, since the lining is gone. This is not always the case, however, and some women end up undergoing a second endometrial ablation or move right along to have a hysterectomy because of continued bleeding. Fibroids play a key role in this and if intramural or subserosal fibroids are present, you may want to consider another method of reducing or eliminating your abnormal bleeding. For instance, if you do not have intramural fibroids but DO have subserosal fibroids, you might want to consider combining myolysis with endometrial ablation. There is some research to indicate this to be a successful combination for many women. In this case, you are treating not only the symptom of bleeding but also the fibroids through a slightly more invasive procedure.

While endometrial ablation does seem to be an effective means of treating abnormal bleeding, it is NOT an effective stand-alone treatment for all symptoms related to uterine fibroids.

Anemia, Fatigue

Anemia is the direct result of an abnormal decrease in the body's red blood cells. If you have passed a lot of blood lately, you may be anemic as a result.

Red blood cells work to keep hemoglobin healthy. Hemoglobin is the protein that carries oxygen from the lungs to the tissues. There's a bit of a balancing act here in how this all works together with iron to get your body the oxygen it needs. When you lose a lot of blood, the body adapts by adding water to the circulating blood volume. This, in turn, causes less and less oxygen-filled hemoglobin to be circulated and eventually results in oxygen starvation.

In an effort to get more oxygen, your heart is forced to pump harder and faster than normal. In the meantime, all your other organs need oxygen, too, and your body attempts to determine which organs need oxygen the least in order to preserve itself and survive. Generally, your skin loses out first, which is why anemic, light-skinned people look extremely pale. Your kidneys are the very next organs in line to receive reduced oxygen flow. Other side effects of anemia are:

➤ shortness of breath
➤ fatigue
➤ dizziness/fainting
➤ ringing in the ears
➤ headaches
➤ dimmed vision
➤ loss of appetite
➤ nausea
➤ constipation
➤ heart failure

So what in the world can you do about anemia? First off, a simple blood test will determine whether or not you are anemic. If your hemoglobin is less than 12.0 g/dL (12 grams of hemoglobin for 1 deciliter of whole blood), then you are anemic. A hemoglobin of 10 to 12 g/dL is mild anemia; between 7 and 10 g/dL is moderate anemia; and anything less than 7 g/dL is severe anemia. Severe anemia *may* require blood transfusions.

After anemia is confirmed, your doctor may direct you to take iron supplementation. Iron combines to work with hemoglobin in storing and transporting oxygen throughout your body. Without iron, hemoglobin cannot exist. Iron supplementation brings about an increase in blood hemoglobin that gets things back on track.

Blood loss and subsequent anemia are two primary symptoms that you need to keep an eye on and work closely with your doctor to control as much as possible. Fibroids can suck the life out of you all right. Lack of hemoglobin and subsequent lack of oxygen flowing through your body are major hindrances to even getting out of bed in the morning. Don't ignore these serious symptoms!

Chronic Pelvic and/or Back Pain and Pressure

With the growth of uterine fibroids, space in your abdomen quickly begins to fill. Fibroids grow in every direction, shape, and size and settle into your pelvic region in ways that are truly unimaginable. Pain? Pressure? The bigger they get, the worse it becomes. Fibroids distort your spine, put pressure on other organs, and eventually start to make you look downright pregnant. Indeed, women with particularly large or protruding fibroids will sometimes nickname their fibroids and talk about them using labels such as "Junior," "Puppy," or "My Little Fruit Basket," much as Marie did when her fibroid uteri grew to thirty weeks in size: *"I'm not feeling so upbeat this morning. I'm soooo tired, extremely depressed, and have to literally force myself to eat. I will be so glad when this is over. 'Junior' misbehaved again, so I had to sleep with the heating pad all night."*

While most fibroids don't really weigh a lot, some can grow to weigh what seems like a ton, but probably weigh only 2 to 5 pounds. Fibroids that are in a size range of over a twenty-week pregnancy may weigh over ten pounds. Excessive abdominal weight can, in turn, put quite a strain on your back. Think bowling ball. Think watermelon. Think about the disproportion this presents to your body, the abdominal muscles becoming weaker and weaker trying to keep it all in place, and your back straining hard to keep you standing upright.

If you are currently experiencing this much discomfort, it's critical that you start considering the options identified in chapter 6, ***Treat the Fibroids.***

Pain may be considered "chronic" if it lasts more than a month. If you're experiencing chronic pain or pelvic pressure, you're probably already following the number-one recommendation: taking an over-the-counter drug like Ibuprofen™ or some other NSAID. Be aware that too much of this type of drug can cause additional stomach irritation.

Your doctor may prescribe oral contraceptives in an attempt to alleviate menstrual-related pain, but these may cause you additional problems with water retention and weight gain.

Exercise is almost always a good option to try. With abdominal distortion due to fibroids growing every which way, the muscles that support your fibroid uterus are weakened. This can cause additional stress on your lower back as it attempts to do the job that your abdominal muscles are not capable of handling. Exercise aimed at strengthening the abdominal muscles and lower back can help to alleviate some chronic pain. Of course, if you're experiencing anemia and fatigue, exercise may be too strenuous an option to carry out.

Which moves us right along to . . . psychological counseling. Before you jump off the deep end at this suggestion, let me explain. I'm not sug-

gesting your pain is imaginary or that you need deep psychological counseling to get to the root of your pain. My only assumption in this case is
that fibroids are causing you pain. End of story. Psychological counseling
can be of tremendous benefit in helping you to learn pain-coping techniques. While they may not work for everyone, coping techniques, deep-
breathing exercises, and relaxation techniques can help some women to
gain control over the chronic pain they feel.

Pain Mapping

Although all the items discussed in the previous paragraphs in this section are ways in which you may be able to treat or learn to cope with the
pain you experience from uterine fibroids, it's important to point out that
chronic pelvic pain can stem from health issues other than fibroids. In
fact, chronic pelvic pain can be an elusive condition stemming from any
one of a wide number of illnesses. Diagnosis is often frustrating for both
the patient and physician as pinning down the precise cause of pain can
be extremely difficult. There are four major organ systems located in the
pelvic region that may be the source of pain:

➤ gynecologic/reproductive
➤ urologic (urinary system)
➤ gastrointestinal (stomach and intestine)
➤ musculoskeletal (bones, muscles, joints)

Within each of those organ systems, there are a dozen or so potential
causes of pain and it is extremely possible that pain can be generated and
compounded from more than one source. Uterine fibroids are considered
only one of over fifty potential sources of chronic pelvic pain. Fibroids do
not always cause pain and they may very well **not** be the source of your
pain. Communication with your physician about any pelvic pain you are
experiencing is very important. However, doctors and patients alike can
easily become frustrated trying to locate and determine the source of
chronic pelvic pain. Physicians have a seemingly wide range of potential
sources of pain to rule out, while patients have a difficult time communicating through the pain and maintaining patience with their physician's
probing questions (many of which may seem unrelated to the pelvic
pain) and diagnostic tests.

In trying to determine and diagnose the source of your pain, your physician may use a process called "pain mapping." In order to assist your physician in the diagnosis, you can begin the pain mapping process by identifying the primary areas in your body where you experience pain. For instance, do you have low back pain or pain in a specific region of your abdomen? Do you have headaches? Experience leg pain? Identify all locations in your body where pain occurs and log them in a journal. (See *chapter 9* **Keeping a Journal**.)

Next, begin keeping a diary of your symptoms in your journal. Be sure to write down how long the pain lasts, how severe it is, whether medication helps, and anything else that you can think of that might be related to the pain. Rate your pain on a scale of 1 to 10 with 1 representing only mild pain and 10 indicating severe pain.

It may also be a good idea to try to describe the pain in your journal. Is it sharp? Piercing? Pulling? Are there things that make the pain worse or, perhaps, seem to make it better? Additional questions your physician may ask include the following:

➤ Do you experience pain during sex?
➤ Have you ever been physically abused? Sexually abused?
➤ How much sleep are you getting?
➤ How much physical exercise are you getting?
➤ Have you been/or are you depressed? (Depression, as well as other emotional events, can intensify physical pain. This question is not asked simply to determine whether or not the pain is just "all in your head.")
➤ How does the pain interfere with your daily life?
➤ What medications, prescription and/or over-the-counter, or herbal remedies are you taking?

All these questions (and many more) are extremely relevant in your search for answers regarding whatever chronic pelvic pain you may be experiencing. To assist your physician and, perhaps, make diagnosing your source of pain easier on both of you, keep in mind one thing: Nothing is too great or too small to log in your journal and share with your doctor. Nothing. Log it all, share it all, then work *with* your doctor in determining the source of your pain. Appropriate treatment cannot be administered without appropriate diagnosis first.

Constipation

Growing fibroids that put pressure on the rectum frequently cause constipation and hemorrhoids. When fibroids grow on the back side of your uterus (directly placing pressure on your rectum), one thing leads to another and the blood vessels and nerves located there that go into your legs may also be impacted. It's all about circulation, and if your fibroids are pressing back and cutting off circulation, your legs can definitely be in trouble.

Constipation can also be a side effect of taking iron supplementation for anemia. Eating more whole grains, bran, and fruit and drinking lots of water may help alleviate constipation. Natural laxative products containing psyllium fiber (such as Metamucil®) are also useful in alleviating symptoms of constipation. Although this may seem like an embarrassing or even silly symptom to bring up and discuss with your doctor, it is important to do so. While you can certainly buy over-the-counter remedies that are either herbal or synthetic, it's important to remember that you do not want to take a remedy that may be counterproductive to prescribed medications you may be taking.

Urinary Incontinence

Let's face it. With large fibroids competing for space in your abdomen and possibly pressing in on your bladder all the time, urinary incontinence is a polite medical way of saying you're seriously compromised in your ability to control your bladder. In addition to pressure and space competition from the fibroids, your muscles have probably been weakened as well and you may not have the ability to "hold" your urine any longer.

In practical terms, urinary incontinence really means that you're staking out bathrooms everywhere you go and coming awfully close to "wetting your pants" quite frequently. Maybe you do urinate in your pants once in a while, and maybe you've even taken to wearing adult diapers or sanitary napkins all the time—"just in case." This is no fun. Here's a backward glance from a woman who chose to get treatment for her fibroids as she remembered the urinary incontinence that had once ruled her life:

> *Last night I did step aerobics and stayed dry. Before getting treatment, I had to wear a pad and that wasn't even enough. I would still have a mess by the time I was done. I could never go to a gym. I had to do aerobics only at home, unless I wanted to be terribly embarrassed. Last night I made it through the aerobics class . . . nothing leaked out. My fifteen-year-old daughter, who teased me previously because I would wet all over, said, "Mommy is a big girl now!" Anyway, I'm thrilled, I can actually go out and do aerobics with other adults without wearing a Depends™ diaper now.*
> —Penny

What should you do about urinary incontinence? What CAN you do about urinary incontinence? First of all, working with your doctor you need to make sure that other medical conditions like diabetes are not causing your urinary-frequency or incontinence problems. Fibroids create a lot of physical problems but they are not, necessarily, responsible for every symptom you may be experiencing. Working with your doctor on this issue is critical, as you do not want to overlook the possibility of some other serious condition.

If fibroids ARE the cause of your urinary incontinence, there isn't generally a lot you can do about it other than seeking treatment for the fibroids. Practicing Kegal exercises—tensing and releasing the muscles responsible for "holding" your urine and bowel movements—is helpful. But if you haven't been doing them all along, it may not prove beneficial at this stage of the game.

On the other side of the coin, you may feel as if you have to go to the bathroom all the time—but are not able to release much urine once you're actually in the bathroom. This is a troublesome sign that your fibroids are growing too large and possibly blocking the exit pathway of your urine—the urethra. This can be extremely painful as urine backs up and builds pressure in your bladder. You may find yourself in the hospital with a catheter inserted to release this urine.

Fibroids can also press on the ureters—the passage tubes that connect the kidneys to the bladder—and back up urine into the kidneys. At this point, serious kidney damage (hydronephrosis) may result. Forget the "Treat the Symptoms" route. It's definitely time to move on to "Treating the Fibroids."

Six

Treat the Fibroids

This chapter assumes that you: 1) don't want to bother wasting any time trying to treat your fibroid symptoms, 2) are fed up with trying to treat the symptoms, or 3) are beyond all hope and just want "it" over with. "It" in this case, being something, ANYTHING, that will actually treat your fibroids and eliminate the problem altogether. Your fibroids are a major symptomatic problem and you need to take care of them to get your life back. If that's the case, you've come to the right chapter. Each of the procedures currently available for treating uterine fibroids is outlined in this chapter. **Treat the Fibroids** consists of the following treatment options:

1. myomectomy
   - ➤ laparoscopic myomectomy
   - ➤ hysteroscopic myomectomy
   - ➤ laparotomy (abdominal myomectomy)
   - ➤ laparoscopic myomectomy with mini-laparotomy
   - ➤ laparoscopic-assisted vaginal myomectomy (LAVM)
2. uterine artery embolization (UAE)
3. myolysis / cryomyolysis
4. hysterectomy
   - ➤ laparoscopic supracervical hysterectomy (LSH)
   - ➤ (abdominal) supracervical hysterectomy (SH)
   - ➤ laparoscopic-assisted vaginal hysterectomy (LAVH)
   - ➤ total vaginal hysterectomy (TVH)

➤ total abdominal hysterectomy (TAH)
➤ total abdominal hysterectomy with bilateral salpingo-oophorectomy (TAH/BSO)

In addition to all the above treatment options, there are a few additional treatment options that merit some discussion in this chapter.

1. clinical trials/research
2. lupron (gonadotropin-releasing hormones—GnRH)
3. mifepristone (RU-486)
4. female reconstructive surgery (FRS)

For each treatment option, this chapter attempts to describe the procedure, identify what makes up an "ideal patient" for the particular option, detail the successes, failures, and complications, and provide a little
bit of history about each procedure.

Myomectomy

Myomectomy is a surgical procedure to remove uterine fibroids and leave
the uterus intact. Little has been written about myomectomy in the medical literature because fewer than 40,000 are actually performed in the
United States each year: pretty small potatoes compared with hysterectomy. It doesn't help any that the American College of Obstetricians
and Gynecologists (ACOG) recognizes this procedure ONLY for women
who want to have more children. Myomectomy can, however, actually
weaken the uterus, make childbearing more difficult, and make the uterus
more prone to rupture.

For women who experience pain and bulk symptoms from uterine fibroids, myomectomy can be the procedure that saves the day. For others,
the mere thought of walking around with fibroids growing inside is
enough to get them to a surgeon to have them removed. They're benign—but so what?—they're still inside of you and entirely unwanted.
Why should these women have to continue suffering or undergo a hysterectomy when they simply want their fibroids out? They shouldn't. Myomectomy can take care of the fibroids and allow many woman to keep
her uterus. I do mean, by the way, ANY woman. At ANY age.

Postmenopausal women who choose to take hormone replacement therapy with estrogen can suddenly find fibroids growing again. They made it to menopause, decided to take estrogen to keep the hormones in balance, and now they have to deal with growing fibroids. To top it all off, they get age discrimination shoved at them when they try to find a doctor who'll simply remove the fibroids. There is no reason whatsoever for these women to be disqualified from a myomectomy. It has no more risk than a hysterectomy—maybe less in a great many cases. If you're a woman who fits this category with uterine fibroids, keep looking—there are doctors out there who do not participate in age discrimination. They understand that a fibroid is a fibroid—regardless of the age of the patient.

Fibroid Growth After Age 60

With age comes increased risk of leiomyosarcoma. While the increase isn't huge, up to 1 percent of women in their 60s and beyond will have a cancerous tumor instead of a benign uterine fibroid. If you are post menopausal and begin experiencing unusual bleeding accompanied with sudden growth of fibroids, it's important to be checked for the potential of cancer.

Myomectomy Procedures

There are three primary ways that doctors perform a myomectomy. The type, size, and location of your fibroids determine which of the following myomectomies might be recommended.

1. laparoscopic myomectomy
2. hysteroscopic myomectomy
3. laparotomy (abdominal myomectomy)

In short, laparoscopic myomectomy is the removal of pedunculated subserosal fibroids through the belly button; hysteroscopic myomectomy is for submucosal fibroids that can be removed vaginally; and laparotomy takes care of all fibroids no matter their location, size, or number.

In addition to these three methods of myomectomy, there are two additional types of myomectomies that are actually a combination of surgical techniques allowing for the removal of slightly larger fibroids without a full laparotomy:

4. laparoscopic myomectomy with mini-laparotomy
5. laparoscopic assisted vaginal myomectomy (LAVM)

Laparoscopic Myomectomy Through use of a laparoscope, this type of myomectomy removes pedunculated subserosal fibroids and small subserosal fibroids not growing too deeply into the uterus. During the procedure, the fibroids are chopped up and suctioned out through the laparoscope, which requires only a small abdominal incision. Usually women experience very little discomfort and pain, and are up and around fairly quickly after the procedure. Without a large abdominal incision, the complication and infection rates are much lower and the total recovery time is only a few days to a week or so.

The biggest drawback? It's not always a piece of cake. Sometimes the doctor has to switch over to laparotomy. He might not be able to see everything or safely maneuver your uterus to remove your fibroids through the laparoscope. If the subserosal fibroids are growing too deeply into the uterus and the surgeon attempts to remove them with the laparoscope, excessive bleeding can occur. A laparotomy would be necessary to stop the bleeding and repair the uterus.

Not all gynecologists do laparoscopic myomectomy or do it well. Many doctors won't recommend this type of myomectomy if their skill level is insufficient. Unfortunately, they won't refer you to someone else who IS more skilled either. They'll push for either a laparotomy or hysterectomy instead. This is one of those times when it's absolutely critical for you to know about your fibroids. What kind of fibroids do you have, how many are there, where are they located? You can control, to some degree, the type of recommendation that is made for you when you demonstrate to the doctor that you have knowledge of your condition and you know what the appropriate recommendations *should* be. If you think laparoscopic myomectomy is an appropriate treatment option for your fibroids and find it isn't being recommended, ask why. Your doctor may have a very legitimate reason for recommending laparotomy instead. In that case, it is still appropriate to find out what that reason might be.

Hysteroscopic Myomectomy Hysteroscopic myomectomy involves placing a hysteroscope into the uterus by going up through the vagina and cervical canal to view your submucosal fibroids. Any fibroids that are definitely visible through this avenue to your uterus can usually be removed with an instrument called the resectoscope. Your doctor might tell you he is "resecting" your submucosal fibroids. The resectoscope is a special instrument designed to destroy unwanted tissue invading the uterine lining. Not all submucosal fibroids can be removed with this technique, however. If the fibroids are large or growing broadly across the endometrium and the surgeon attempts to remove them with the hysteroscope, excessive bleeding can occur. Should this happen, a laparotomy would be necessary to stop the bleeding and repair the uterus.

Most of the time this procedure is done under general anesthesia. It's typically performed on an "outpatient" basis, as it usually takes no more than sixty minutes to complete and involves only a few hours of recovery time.

Hysteroscopic myomectomy is a fairly safe procedure, with complications occurring less than 1 percent of the time. Remember though, only 5 percent of all fibroids are submucosal. Pat yourself on the back if you're one of the lucky women who only have submucosal fibroids—preferably pedunculated for easier removal!

Laparotomy (Abdominal Myomectomy) The only thing you can do for intramural fibroids to remove them (and leave the uterus) is a laparotomy. But look on the bright side—if you happen to have a "fruit basket" of fibroids in and on your uterus, you can be rid of them with one procedure. Of course, with a laparotomy the surgery is much more difficult and requires an abdominal incision. Because of this, the complication and infection rate does go up a bit. So does the blood transfusion rate, since this is a major abdominal surgery to remove all your fibroids. That may mean quite a bit of cutting, removing, and repairing of the layers of tissue that are spread open with an incision during this procedure.

Because of the abdominal incision, this procedure generally requires a short hospital stay of around three days. After that, it's another four weeks or so before you're completely healed and ready to go back out and conquer the world.

> "I wanted this procedure but I couldn't find a gynecologist who would do it. Every single doctor that I consulted told me that my large, pedunculated, subserosal fibroid was better served with a hysterectomy. I knew better than that. But it didn't really matter because finding a doctor who would do a myomectomy on a woman who was done with her "childbearing" years was impossible. One can only hope that time and medical advances in science change that kind of thinking in the gynecological community soon."
> —Sandy

Laparoscopic Myomectomy with Mini-Laparotomy This technique allows for the removal of slightly larger submucosal fibroids than what the laparoscope alone can handle and generally includes a relatively small incision of three inches or less in the abdomen.

Laparoscopic Assisted Vaginal Myomectomy (LAVM) This technique is not performed by the vast majority of gynecologists but does allow for the laparoscopic removal of subserosal fibroids from the uterus with the total removal of fibroid material through an incision in the vagina. While this does allow for the removal of slightly larger subserosal fibroids without an abdominal incision, the vaginal incision created has increased risks for infection and poor wound healing. Even so, some gynecologists are reporting good outcome from their patients who undergo this procedure as opposed to the full laparotomy that would have been required due to the size of their subserosal fibroids.

Ideal Patient

The American College of Obstetricians and Gynecologists (ACOG) has developed guidelines to determine who and under what circumstances a woman should have a myomectomy when uterine fibroids are present. Basically, their guidelines indicate that myomectomy should be performed when infertility is an issue and you have not been able to get pregnant or hold on to a pregnancy because of the presence of uterine fibroids. That's it. Since ACOG recognizes no other treatment option for uterine fibroids when they are symptomatic other than hysterectomy, if you don't happen to want a hysterectomy, you are just plain out of luck because myomectomy is for women who want to get pregnant. Well, not exactly.

Even though it is not explicitly outlined within the ACOG guidelines, many gynecologists will perform a myomectomy when the patient chooses to keep her uterus for reasons other than future pregnancy. So, under those circumstances, the ideal patient for this procedure meets three basic requirements:

1. She has fibroids.
2. The fibroids are symptomatic.
3. There is no cancer.

I Said Myomectomy—Not Hysterectomy!

If you are undergoing a myomectomy and you do not want to wake up without your uterus, you must put it in **writing** that you do **not** want a hysterectomy under any circumstances other than those necessary to save your life. Specific instructions to the physicians should be noted on the hospital admitting forms as well as the informed consent document for surgery.

Success, Failures, and Complications

Where uterine fibroids are concerned, success with myomectomy varies depending upon the size, type, and number of fibroids present and the type of myomectomy performed.

Complications and complication rates also vary depending upon the size, type, and number of fibroids present as well as the type of myomectomy performed. In addition to a minor inherent risk of death (much as that with any medical procedure), the following items are considered potential risks of myomectomy.

1. **Blood Transfusion.** If a severe blood loss occurs during or after the procedure, a blood transfusion may be necessary. This occurs approximately 20 to 30 percent of the time. In addition, if this occurs during laparoscopic or hysteroscopic myomectomy, an exploratory laparotomy (abdominal incision) may be necessary to repair a damaged blood vessel.

About Excessive Bleeding . . .

During the discussion of potential complications you have with your gynecologist, the potential need for blood transfusion will most certainly come up. There are two things that are important to ask:

1. Can you donate your own blood in advance of the surgery so that it can be used if a transfusion becomes necessary (*autologous* blood donation)?
2. Has your gynecologist ever worked with an interventional radiologist (IR) in any cases where excessive bleeding has occurred?

IRs have been performing uterine artery embolization for over twenty years now to stem the tide of excessive bleeding after childbirth or other pelvic surgery. If excessive bleeding during your surgery becomes a problem, an IR is a great doctor to have on call because he can stop the bleeding, reduce the need for emergency hysterectomy, and, quite possibly, save your life. It's not a bad idea to find out whether or not your gynecologist has ever worked with one of these doctors before or is willing to work with one now to ensure that your myomectomy doesn't rapidly convert to a hysterectomy due to excessive bleeding.

---

2. **Damage to Internal Organs.** Accidental injury to internal organs can occur with any form of myomectomy. This might be the result of a perforation or a laceration by an instrument or an electrosurgical

burn. Further surgery may be necessary to repair the organ, which might be done at the time of the procedure or days/weeks after the surgery. Reoperation to investigate uncontrolled hemorrhage or to repair bladder, bowel, or ureteral injuries is necessary about 1 percent of the time. In addition, up to 3 percent of women will develop some form of urinary complications other than infection.

3. **Adhesion Formation.** After any pelvic or abdominal surgery, scar tissue (adhesions) can form. This may result in abdominal or pelvic pain, or intestinal obstruction.
4. **Postoperative.** Infection may develop at the site of surgery or elsewhere, and may require antibiotics. It may also result in additional surgery. Severe infections after laparoscopic or hysteroscopic myomectomy surgery are uncommon.
5. **Ureter Damage.** Up to 1 percent may be damaged due to laceration, inadvertent binding of the ureter (ligation), compression, or puncture. Reoperation may be required to repair ureter damage.
6. **Blood Clots.** Rare but potentially deadly. Typically form in the legs but can travel to the lungs or brain.

In addition to those complications, there are a couple of additional factors that contribute to the overall, long-term failure of a myomectomy. If you are undergoing myomectomy in the hope of simply stopping excessive bleeding (possibly due to submucosal fibroids), you should know that nearly 20 percent of patients do **not** experience a decrease in bleeding. There are many reasons for developing menorrhagia (excessive bleeding) in the first place, and fibroids are only one of those reasons. If excessive bleeding continues after the removal of your fibroids, it's important to continue working with your gynecologist to attempt to diagnose a cause and obtain appropriate treatment.

The other item that contributes to the long-term failure of myomectomy is simply that fibroids continue to develop and grow in your uterus. You have them removed, but more grow in. As long as the hormonal imbalance that caused the fibroids to develop in the first place is still happening in your body, the likelihood that fibroids will continue to grow is pretty good. A lot of women start using progesterone cream or taking some form of prescribed synthetic progesterone about this time, so the hormonal imbalance scale is tipped back a bit.

A second round of fibroid growth after a myomectomy happens about 25 percent of the time but generally requires additional treatment (such as a second myomectomy or a hysterectomy) only 10 percent of the time. Generally, the older you are when you have a myomectomy, the less likely it is that the fibroids will recur or that you will need additional treatment.

History of Myomectomy

The first reported case of a myomectomy was, believe it or not, sometime in the mid to late 1800s. No one really knows who performed the first myomectomy, but a man by the name of Eugene Koeberle was the first to write about the removal of fibroids in 1864. Over time, myomectomy became widely accepted, but the death rate from complications of this procedure remained at around 5 percent until the 1940s. That's right. Five out of every one hundred women died.

Around 1942, Dr. Rubin at Mount Sinai Hospital wrote about a relatively large (for that time) case series of patients who underwent myomectomy. There were 171 patients in the study, and by applying the previous 5 percent death-rate standards at least 9 women should have died. This was the first time, however, that not a single patient died during a study of myomectomy. Back then, patients stayed in the hospital about three weeks to recover from this major abdominal surgery. At least they ALL lived to tell about it.

Money and Myomectomy vs. Hysterectomy

It's been argued that gynecologists make the same income from performing a myomectomy as they do from performing a hysterectomy. Because of this, some doctors believe that gynecologists do not, therefore, have a vested stake in either one of those procedures. In the end, I'm told that women will choose a hysterectomy over a myomectomy—hands down—and that THAT is why the hysterectomy numbers are so high in the United States.

Well, gynecologists may earn the same income from myomectomy, but they certainly don't spend the same amount of time in the surgical suite performing a myomectomy. Isn't time money? Since the complications rate is no worse with myomectomy than it is with hysterectomy, I can only assume that women are "choosing" hysterectomy over myomectomy because that is what they are being "offered" by their doctors. The following is just one example of how some gynecologists paint a myomectomy as a procedure prone to serious complications and, at the same time, paint a hysterectomy as a rather simple procedure without complications.

"I have a rather large size fibroid and I tried to talk to my gyn about having a myomectomy. She would prefer I have hysterectomy. Her reason is that at my age (forty), why not have it done? Especially since I'm not planning on having any more children. If I really, really want to have kids, she will do the myomectomy. But she claims that with a myomectomy there are infections, damage to other organs and a possible need for blood transfusions during the procedure. I think she is trying to scare me into having a hysterectomy . . ."
—Paula

As women become more informed as to the actual complications of BOTH procedures, they are more inclined to simply switch doctors when the above kind of communication takes place.

"I am in the process of finding a new doctor. Any doctor unwilling to train and learn new techniques but VERY willing to terrorize me to promote a treatment I don't want as a lifestyle improvement is a health hazard more than anything else."
—Nancy

Uterine Artery Embolization

Uterine artery embolization (UAE, also known as uterine *fibroid* embolization [*UFE*]) is a noninvasive, nonsurgical procedure performed by an interventional radiologist (IR). In order to do UAE, the IR performs a puncture of the artery in the leg and then inserts a catheter, guiding it to the uterus. The IR then injects a material that is opaque to x-rays in order to outline the arteries. This is called an angiogram. Next, small particles of plastic (polyvinyl alcohol, or **PVA**, embospheres, or gelfoam) are injected into the uterine artery. The particles travel to the fibroids and block the blood supply feeding the fibroids; this results in *embolization.*

The whole procedure takes about an hour and you are sedated but awake the entire time.

Within minutes after the procedure, the fibroids begin dying. Generally, but not always, there is an overnight stay in the hospital because many women have felt intense abdominal cramping and pain.

Post-procedural pain is usually controlled through the use of a combination of narcotics. A patient controlled morphine pump is very common. Some IRs use epidurals or spinal anesthesia to block all pelvic region pain for twelve hours or so. The perfect combination of drugs to control pain with this procedure has not been agreed upon across the board with interventional radiologists, and there is quite a bit of variation in what, exactly, a patient might be given. In addition, allergies and back disorders can have an influence on what kind of medication is ultimately used. Since anesthesia of any kind can add risk to a procedure, it's important to discuss with your doctor all your options for controlling pain brought on by UAE when you meet with him before the procedure.

Ninety-nine percent of the women who undergo this procedure go home after only one night in the hospital. Complete recovery usually takes one to two weeks, but most women are up and around within a couple of days. The majority return to work after only a one-week recovery period.

There have been only rare cases of traumatic outcome from this procedure. Most women experience tremendous amounts of positive feelings almost immediately after recovery from this procedure. Relief at being able to avoid major surgery, such as that with myomectomy or hysterectomy, along with the knowledge that they have undergone a procedure that allows them to retain their uterus, generally seems to override any amount of pain experienced as a result of this procedure.

Ideal Patient

The ideal patient for this procedure meets four basic requirements:

1. She has fibroids.
2. The fibroids are symptomatic.
3. There is no cancer.
4. Future pregnancies are not desired.

A Note about Pain
and Self-Medication . . .

I chose this procedure for treatment of my uterine fibroids and returned to work after only six days of medical leave. But, I probably should have waited and returned after the second week because of post-embolization syndrome symptoms (see box, next page). Even so, there was no traumatic surgery to recover from, no hormonal whammies from having anything "removed," and no psychological stress involved regarding the removal of the uterus.

I did, however, experience a tremendous amount of pain for about 48 hours following this procedure—almost unbearable pain. During the year before undergoing UAE, I suffered a great deal of back pain; and, in an effort to seek relief from this pain, I consumed a lot of pain medication. This information was not disclosed to my physician and, subsequently, he was not aware of my high tolerance to pain medication nor was he prepared for my total lack of relief from the administration of morphine.

If you choose this procedure and are currently taking high doses of medication to numb physical pain, please share this information with your gynecologist and interventional radiologist. It is the only way they can properly prepare for your pain medication needs postprocedure.

Although some interventional radiologists may have additional requirements, it has not been proven yet that any of these requirements have a basis in scientific data collected thus far. For instance, one interventional radiologist states that he doesn't accept patients who have a fibroid uterus that has grown above the navel in size—any fibroid uterus roughly larger than a twenty-week pregnancy is unacceptable. In his experience, the amount of shrinkage that occurs from this size of fibroid uterus is not enough to warrant doing the procedure. However, his experience may include fewer than a dozen patients with fibroids of this size. Collectively, the data simply hasn't been reviewed yet for how effective UAE is in relation to the size of the fibroid uterus. Who knows whether or not his exclusionary patient selection process is valid? Maybe it is. Maybe it isn't.

Postembolization Syndrome

Postembolization syndrome is something that many women have experienced with uterine artery embolization. Although most of the immediate side effects do not last long, postembolization syndrome can take up to six weeks to go away.

So what is this syndrome? It consists mostly of menopause-type symptoms, such as fever, hot flashes, a general sense of not feeling well, and nausea. It can be downright annoying and troublesome.

As the fibroids die, toxins are released into the bloodstream that can cause these symptoms. While the majority of women recover from these symptoms within one to two weeks postprocedure, they have been known to last as long as six weeks.

CRITICAL NOTE: If any of the symptoms you experience include an ever-increasing amount of pain or a rise in fever above 100.5° that does not subside within a short period of time, this may be due to an infection. *Contact your physician immediately for further evaluation.*

Still other IRs are turning women away because they are fifty years of age or more. Since the average age of menopause is fifty-one, they've somehow determined that doing nothing and simply waiting out menopause is a more appropriate course to take for these women. Well, maybe it is. On the other hand, they are not taking into consideration that fifty-one is the *average* age of menopause. (*The women in my family didn't hit menopause by the age of fifty-one!*) Women in their fifties can be bleeding like there's no tomorrow just like younger women and, quite possibly, be a good five years or more away from menopause. If there is any question whatsoever about whether or not a woman is postmenopausal, there are certainly diagnostic tests that can be performed to confirm the levels of FSH (follicle stimulating hormones) and LH (luteinizing hormones) in her system.

The average age of menopause is fifty-one, give or take one to fifteen years.

Regardless of whether or not a woman has reached menopause, it is still possible for excessive bleeding to occur with uterine fibroids. Under these circumstances and with the ruling out of any cancerous conditions, there is every reason to believe that this bleeding could be helped with uterine artery embolization.

Some additional concerns and considerations might include:

➤ the presence of submucosal fibroids, which can or should be removed with a hysteroscopic myomectomy
➤ the presence of pedunculated subserosal fibroids more effectively treated by removing them with myomectomy

UAE treats all uterine fibroids at the same time and is, therefore, an extremely effective, all-encompassing treatment option. However, submucosal fibroids not removed before UAE may create problems once they die—causing the uterus to attempt to get rid of the fibroid. If the fibroid is too large for the uterus to pass through the cervical canal, serious infection could result. This can be extremely painful and potentially dangerous. It is important for women with submucosal fibroids to discuss this possibility with their gynecologist and determine how to handle the care of their submucosal fibroids *before* the UAE.

Pedunculated subserosal fibroids may also cause problems by breaking off from the uterus once they completely die. This has been known to create a temporarily painful condition treatable with pain medication but, so far, no additional problems have been encountered. Only more time will tell us whether or not this is a complication with additional concerns.

Success, Failures, and Complications

Doctors are currently tracking success and failure of this procedure by two different standards: **technical failure** and **clinical failure.** Knowing the difference between these two kinds of failures will give you a better understanding of what the success statistics actually mean to you when you read them. In addition, **complications** can occur during the procedure that result in injury, a less than desired outcome, or unanticipated results.

Technical Failure Rates Technical failure, the inability to complete the procedure as planned or without technical difficulties, currently occur 1 to 2 percent of the time and are primarily related to the following factors:

1. Skill of the interventional radiologist.
2. Abnormalities of the uterine artery (increase the difficulty of completing the procedure).

3. Shared blood flow from a single uterine artery and ovarian artery where both feed the fibroids. This is a blood flow situation called *anastomoses* which makes it impossible to embolize the uterine artery without impacting the ovarian artery.
4. Use of progestin or GnRH agonists (for example, Lupron) pre-UAE, which causes the blood vessels to be more constricted and difficult to navigate with the catheter.
5. Any number of additional odd circumstances that present themselves during the procedure.

Clinical Failure Rates Clinical failure rates are another cup of tea entirely. Typically, these have nothing to do with the interventional radiologist and his embolization of your artery but rather your own physical response to the embolization. If the embolization is a technical success (all went well during the procedure with none of the above-identified factors related to technical failures creating a problem) but the symptoms the fibroids were causing are not significantly or satisfactorily reduced after the UAE, then this is considered a clinical failure. For example, if the fibroids don't shrink "enough" or excessive bleeding doesn't subside, then the UAE could be considered a clinical failure.

You won't see the term *clinical failure rates* in medical literature, however. Instead, you'll see numbers that tout the statistics of how many women report "shrinkage" or reduced bleeding. Like this:

"... *80 to 90 percent of all women undergoing UAE report* ..."

Sort of "reverse statistics" to get you to focus on the positive side of things. Here's the reality: 80 to 90 percent success rates equal a 10 to 20 percent failure. **10 to 20 percent clinical failure rate.** (Some IRs report 10 to 15 percent and others 15 to 20 percent.) The numbers look different to you now, don't they? 10 to 20 percent of all women undergoing UAE will not experience success in fibroid shrinkage and/or in getting their bleeding under control.

Here's something the numbers won't tell you:

Even with high clinical failure rates, women (even those who were considered to have clinical failure) are reporting that they would STILL choose UAE over hysterectomy or even myomectomy if they had it to do all over again.

Why is that? Why do women who've had "less than success" with their UAE still perceive it to be a better option? From my own personal experience, I would say it's because even though the procedure wasn't a *complete* success, it was enough to restore life to an acceptable level of existence—and, at minimal surgical (technical) risk, particularly compared to hysterectomy or even myomectomy.

Complications Significant complications currently occur 1 to 2 percent of the time. **Fewer than 1 in 200 women will acquire an infection that requires an immediate hysterectomy.** Other factors that contribute to the complication rate are:

1. Finding that the woman has only **a single uterine artery and the ovarian artery is feeding the fibroids.** In some cases, the uterine artery may be feeding the ovary since the blood can actually flow in either direction. The angiogram images of the uterine arteries tell the IR if there is a significant supply of blood to the fibroids coming from the ovarian arteries. Since this imaging is done at the time of catheterization of the arteries, it is impossible to know the blood flow situation of the uterine and ovarian arteries before the embolization is in process. This shared blood flow is called *anastomoses.* Doctors do one of two things in this case:
   ➤ partially embolize the ovarian artery (which may cause premature menopause)
   ➤ proceed with embolizing the uterine artery. In this case, the fibroids continue to receive blood from the ovarian artery so the overall amount of "shrinkage" to the fibroids is reduced significantly. However, if the blood is actually flowing to the ovaries from the uterus, embolization will shut off the blood supply to the ovaries causing instant menopause.

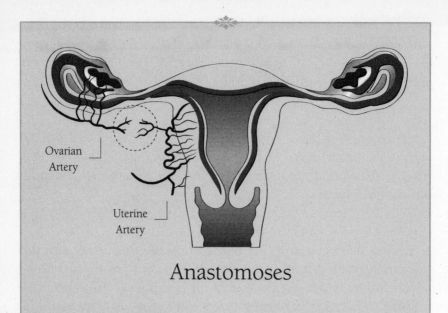

Ovarian
Artery

Uterine
Artery

Anastomoses

This illustration is representative of only one way in which anastomoses occurs. In reality, there are many ways in which the blood can be shared or compromised between the ovarian artery and the uterine artery. In this particular example, the shared blood flow occurs at an "in-between" location entirely separate from both the uterus and the ovary. If the direction of the blood flow were **from** the ovary to the uterus, embolizing only the uterine artery would not stop that blood flow to the fibroids, and they would continue to receive blood from the ovarian artery.

On the other hand, if the blood is actually flowing from the uterine artery to the ovarian artery, then embolizing the uterine artery may result in a decreased blood flow to the ovary—possibly causing reduced functioning of the ovary or complete menopause.

2. Complete **misembolization of the ovarian artery.** Could result in menopause, amenorrhea, and/or infertility.
3. **Misembolization** of other areas that were not "targeted." In a worst-case scenario, this might, for example, impact your buttocks or legs, possibly even your bladder or bowel. This may also cause sciatic nerve injury. Effect of misembolization are generally temporary but can be quiet serious, depending on what, exactly, the doctor misembolized. Although not reported in the medical literature, there have

been cases of quite serious misembolization. In one case, the buttocks area was embolized and the patient felt a form of paralysis in that region for about six months. In another, much more serious case, the bladder was impacted and the patient required pelvic reconstructive surgery. While these complications are truly rare, it is important to be aware that they can occur.

Misembolization

This complication is typically referred to as **nontarget embolization** in medical literature. I prefer the term *misembolization,* but several interventional radiologists have pointed out to me that this implies there's been a **mis-**take when, in fact, there was simply an embolization of something nontargeted and it could have been a mistake or simply materials going somewhere that they shouldn't have. It's a finer point to make and argue over—one that I think is rather dubious for the doctors to be making. Hey—something got embolized that shouldn't have. End of story. **Misembolization.**

---

4. **Femoral hematoma.** A deep bruising of the puncture site in the groin where the catheter was inserted into the artery.

5. **Death.** While there have been no deaths reported in the United States from UAE, there have been one death in England and a second one in Italy associated with UAE. Statistically, this represents a tiny fraction of the worldwide total number of women (over 10,500 as of November 2000, according to the director of research for the Society of Cardiovascular and International Radiology, Wendy Landow) who have undergone this procedure to date. nonetheless, it is a potential complication of any medical procedure.

6. **Miscellaneous side effects and risks.** Doctors are still figuring these out as they are so infrequent that only time and long-range data collection will give them a more complete list. This list might include: an allergic reaction to dyes or materials, groin infection, *kidney failure, vascular damage,* and *pulmonary embolism.* There is always the small chance that cancer can occur in organs that might otherwise be removed through some other surgical option. Also, since the particles used with embolization are permanently implanted material, there is an

unknown possibility of complications appearing after many years. (So far, with over twenty years of using gelfoam and polyvinyl alcohol particles, complications developing from this implanted material have never been reported.) Ask your interventional radiologist for a more complete list of complication possibilities during your initial appointment.

One of the side effects of UAE may well be some level of **sexual dysfunction.** If you are a woman who experiences uterine contractions or internal pelvic orgasms during sex and the blood flow to the cervix is altered because of uterine artery embolization, you *may* experience a loss of those contractions or internal orgasms.

Although most women are reluctant to discuss this with their physician, there are a number of cases where loss of internal orgasms and/or uterine contractions has, in fact, occurred. Some of these women have passed the one-year mark after UAE and have shown no signs of improvement. There is some speculation that embolizing the cervical branch of the uterine artery may have contributed to this outcome, and some IRs are now attempting to bypass this branch and embolize the uterine artery beyond this point.

Clitoral orgasms and "feelings" in the vagina have also been reported as less intense with some women post UAE, but in most cases these have returned to their previous state within three to six months. Until more women choose to openly discuss the issue of sex with their physicians both before and after UAE, we will not know how often sexual dysfunction actually occurs as a result of this procedure. If sexual function is a concern of yours, do not hesitate to bring up this topic with your gynecologist or interventional radiologist.

Death and UAE

The following are the details involved in the very first published incident of death that occurred as a result of uterine artery embolization for fibroids. Since this is such a new use (of an old procedure), interventional radiologists are showing a fair amount of due diligence in reporting and publishing as many side effects as are noted—including death. Of course, gynecologists wanted to get this information out to the patient population as quickly as possible as well. Complications this severe that can occur with a procedure are important for the medical community to know about. By quickly sharing this information, doctors can analyze the case and come up with ways to avoid such complications in the future.

The woman in this case was fifty-one years old with a two-year history of increasing blood loss due to submucosal fibroids. Doctors were not able to do a hysteroscopic resection, and the woman did not want a hysterectomy. She attempted to use Zoladax (a gonadotropin releasing hormone analogue) to shrink her fibroids—but she suffered severe headaches and eventually stopped taking that drug. Ultimately, she lost so much blood that she required blood transfusions.

She underwent UAE in January 1999 with a fibroid uterus that measured 14 by 12 by 11 centimeters. There were no immediate complications, and she seemed to recover well from the procedure. She did, however, develop a urinary tract infection. She was released from the hospital on antibiotics and oral analgesics. Seven days later she was readmitted with abdominal pain, diarrhea, and vomiting. She had a submucosal fibroid that had "died" and detached itself from her uterus, but it was simply too large for her body to expel through the cervix on its own. Ultimately, she underwent total abdominal hysterectomy and bilateral salpingo-oophorectomy. Nonetheless, after fifteen days in the intensive-care unit, she ultimately died of sepsis (blood poisoning) resulting in multiorgan failure.

For women who are concerned about their own situation and potential for this to occur to them, it can never be understated that it is important for each and every one of us to actively participate in our medical care by obtaining as much information as possible about our condition. Know what kind of uterine fibroids you have, where they are located, how large they are, and ALL your potential options for treating them. Learn about the potential risks regarding your particular type of fibroids (as different types of fibroids carry different risks and different treatment options) so that you can be proactive in following up with your own recovery process with whatever course of treatment you choose.

Fertility and UAE

Because of the very real potential for any one of the following conditions to occur, most interventional radiologists do NOT recommend uterine artery embolization for women wishing to retain their fertility for future childbirth except under special circumstances.

1. anastomoses (shared blood flow from uterine to ovarian artery or vice versa—results in embolization of the ovary and menopause OR leads to possible failure of the UAE to treat the fibroids)
2. misembolization of ovarian artery (resulting in menopause)
3. infection requiring hysterectomy
4. complete necrosis (death) of the uterus (resulting in hysterectomy)
5. "problems" with the endometrium (possibly reduced blood flow) that interfere with implantation of eggs
6. uterine rupture during a term pregnancy (loss of baby AND uterus)
7. onset of menopause prematurely for unknown/unidentified causes (possibly reduced blood flow to the ovaries)

Yes, these are all very real *potential* consequences of uterine artery embolization. Conditions 1 through 3 have already occurred and are well documented. Conditions 4 through 7 are all theoretically possible but haven't actually been documented as having occurred yet. Please keep in mind that information on incidents such as those listed above are not always openly shared *or* published. (Actually, this is a true statement regardless of the medical procedure involved. Not all complications are readily reported by physicians.)

Uterine rupture resulting in hysterectomy has occurred. The case involved an infarcted (dead) fibroid that broke off from the uterus. The woman was not pregnant at the time. As it stands, until such a case is *officially* reported, it can only be *speculated* that uterine rupture is a *possibility* during a term pregnancy post UAE.

Early onset of menopause is also troublesome in terms of fertility because it has been reported in Europe that as many as 10 percent of women undergoing UAE have entered into menopause within one year post procedure. Researchers in the United States are now reporting a "rough" figure of 5 percent. However, more long-term studies are required to determine whether this is truly a collateral result of the UAE or a natural occurrence due to the age of women undergoing this procedure—primarily those over the age of thirty-five.

Nonetheless, glowing reports on fertility retention with UAE have been published and broadcast on television. Rarely are potential complications mentioned. Yes, there have been a dozen or so successful pregnancies and the women this has happened to are, by and large, ecstatic. But there have also been hysterectomies, miscarriages, and menopause.

If you are hoping to become pregnant, before walking down the UAE path you may want to consider the risks very carefully and compare them against the risks of other procedures for treatment of your uterine fibroids. In addition, you might want to consider the use of gelfoam instead of polyvinyl alcohol particles as this embolic material has been *speculated* as showing *potentially* less permanence and *possibly* bears less risk when it comes to preventing pregnancy entirely over the remainder of your childbearing years. This speculation is based on experience with gelfoam during the past twenty years where it was used as the embolization material during emergency embolizations resulting from childbirth or surgical hemorrhage. Also, published medical literature on subsequent pregnancies following these emergency embolizations is limited but does exist.

History of UAE

There have been thousands of UAEs performed over the last ten years for the specific treatment of uterine fibroids. Prior to that, this procedure was reserved for women who began hemorrhaging after childbirth or during or after pelvic surgery (such as myomectomy).

Overall, UAE is a procedure that has been documented in the medical literature as an effective means of stopping uncontrollable bleeding since 1979 or so. (Although the Society of Cardiovascular and Interventional Radiology recently changed the name of this procedure to represent its specific treatment application for uterine fibroids, technically UAE and UFE are the same procedure.)

About ten years ago (1989), an obstetrical gynecologist in Paris, France—Dr. Jacques-Henri Ravina—became aware of UAE as an effective means of stopping uncontrollable bleeding and decided to start sending his patients for UAE prior to their myomectomy surgery to cut down on the bleeding that they would experience during the procedure. He was quite surprised to start finding women canceling out on their

Who Was the First?

Leslie Miles (a resident of Hawaii) was the first woman to give birth in the United States following the specific use of uterine artery embolization for the treatment of uterine fibroids. She did not seek out embolization because she wanted additional children—she sought it out because she was looking for an alternative to hysterectomy. She was completely unaware that she could still become pregnant after embolization. Imagine her surprise at finding out she was pregnant!

On February 2, 1997, Dr. Harold Mitty (New York) submitted a case review of twelve women who had undergone emergency UAE between 1990 and 1995. He specifically looked at the impact of UAE on menses and pregnancy and reported three women as having conceived post UAE.

Jacques Ravina (Paris, France) "officially" reported the results of his 1993-plus studies on uterine artery embolization on July 28, 1997, and it was subsequently published in *La Press Medicale* in France on February 21, 1998. As part of that paper he reported four patients who became pregnant. Two miscarried, one had twins via c-section, and one gave birth to a full-term normal baby. All were born prior to July 2, 1997—the date his paper was accepted for publication. Most likely, these babies were the first born in the *world* following the specific use of uterine artery embolization for the treatment of uterine fibroids.

But are these REALLY the first babies born after their mothers underwent uterine artery embolization?

Uterine artery embolization has been around for over twenty years and there are many undocumented, unreported cases of pregnancy that have occurred post UAE; probably hundreds—maybe more. It would be impossible to determine who, exactly, was the first baby born after uterine artery embolization at this time.

myomectomies. They no longer needed the myomectomy because their bleeding had subsided and their fibroids had actually begun to shrink.

From there, it took another seven years before the procedure was introduced into the United States by Dr. Scott Goodwin at the UCLA Medical Center. Since introducing this procedure in 1996, there have been over 10,500 uterine artery embolizations performed (these numbers are current through November 2000). Nonetheless, it has been an uphill struggle to get gynecologists to recognize this promising procedure in the United States.

There is a tremendous amount of speculation as to why gynecologists are hesitant to recognize UAE as a viable option for their patients with little agreement and even less advancement in terms of getting these two medical specialties together to talk it out and work together. Many gynecologists and interventional radiologists have found ways to work together as a team and effectively manage patients who choose to undergo UAE. However, even more gynecologists have simply refused to participate in any aspect of this procedure.

Perhaps these gynecologists simply believe gynecological technologies to be superior and more definitive in terms of treatment for fibroids. Perhaps they believe they are protecting their patients from a relatively little known procedure. Or maybe, just maybe, there is financial motivation behind not recognizing interventional radiology techniques and not choosing, therefore, to refer patients for UAE. There is little doubt that UAE does indeed cut directly into the revenue gynecologists receive from performing a hysterectomy.

On Gynecologists and Money . . .

Many a gynecologist has written to me indicating that they do not believe that gynecologists are refusing to refer patients for UAE based on loss of revenue from not performing a hysterectomy. The debate certainly leaves a lot of questions in my mind. A woman's reproductive organs are clearly on the auction block of medicine in this country. If gynecologists would get busy doing some REAL research on sparing the uterus with uterine fibroid treatments, they might be a little more believable in their protests. No matter how many refinements of a hysterectomy one comes up with, it's important to understand that *it is still a hysterectomy*! Apparently that is a point missed by many gynecologists.

Myolysis/Cryomyolysis

In Myolysis, surgical instruments are inserted through tiny, laparoscopic incisions in the abdomen and, using a special probe, a high-frequency electrical current is sent to the fibroid. The electrical current causes the blood vessels to vaso-constrict (become very small or close down), and this basically cuts off the blood flow to the fibroids. The fibroids remain in place and are not surgically removed. Without a blood supply, the fibroids eventually die and shrink, just as they do with uterine artery embolization.

Cryomyolysis is a similar procedure that "freezes" the fibroids to death. Liquid nitrogen at minus 180 degrees Celsius is applied through a cryoprobe while the doctor monitors the freezing process using ultrasound. Because of the extremely high expense of the equipment required for this procedure, it is rarely performed.

In order to maximize the potential shrinkage that results from this procedure, the patient is usually requested to undergo GnRH therapy for three to six months before the procedure. The goal is to shrink the fibroids by about 50 percent to make the procedure easier to perform. This also gives the patient a better "starting point" for her fibroids to shrink from with the myolysis or cryomyolysis procedure.

Both procedures take about one hour (thirty to ninety minutes), and the patient is observed in the recovery room for approximately another three hours and then discharged to go home. Total recovery from this procedure takes about one week.

Postprocedural Concerns

After returning home from this procedure, if you experience any increase in vaginal bleeding, abdominal pain, swelling, fever, or any other symptoms that are worrisome to you, contact your doctor immediately.

Lupron: A Few Words of Caution

There are many potential side effects to this drug, which was originally developed and FDA approved for the treatment of advanced prostate cancer in men. These days, however, Lupron is widely used by gynecologists to treat women for a variety of routine gynecological problems.

According to a special report series published by the *Boston Herald* in August 1999, some specialists are now saying that the long-term effects of Lupron can be dangerous and harmful, and that not enough studies have been done to adequately demonstrate that it is safe and effective.

As with any other potential treatment option available for your uterine fibroids, it is important to weigh the risks and benefits of potential outcome for each option against your own specific condition, belief system, and overall need for resolution of your situation. Lupron has helped many women. It has also hurt many women. Only **you** can weigh what potential benefit you might receive or not receive from its use and what risks you are willing to take or not take in the pursuit of treating your uterine fibroids.

Ideal Patient

The ideal patient for this procedure meets seven basic requirements:

1. She has subserosal fibroids.
2. The fibroids are symptomatic.
3. The fibroids are within the correct size range.
4. She is willing to take Lupron for several months prior to undergoing this procedure.
5. There is no cancer.
6. She does not desire future pregnancies.
7. She is actively menstruating.

According to Dr. Herbert Goldfarb, a Fellow member of ACOG, neither myolysis nor cryomyolysis can be performed on very large fibroids (anything over 10 cm before Lupron is taken is considered "very large"), nor can either of these procedures be performed if there are more than four fibroids each with a volume of up to 5 cm apiece. Also, anything less than 3 cm in size is too small. In other words:

➤ Fibroids that are too large complicate the procedure and end up shrinking less in the long run.
➤ Bulk-related symptoms may not be resolved when the size of the fibroid at the time of the procedure is still very large. Hence, the use of Lupron.
➤ Too many fibroids may make the amount of time it takes to perform the procedure impossible.
➤ Fibroids less than 3 cm are simply too small to effectively do this procedure.

Bedtime Story . . .

Deciding what size of fibroids can be treated with myolysis or cryomyolysis kind of sounds like the story of The Three Bears, doesn't it? Fibroids can be classified as Papa Bear, Mama Bear, or Baby Bear. Only in this case the fibroids that are "just right" can only be assessed by Goldilocks, err, I mean, your gynecologist. The "ideal size" is probably Mama Bear—but only if there are not too many of them.

Successes, Failures, and Complications

It usually takes between three and six months to determine whether this surgery has been successful. It takes this long before the maximum amount of fibroid shrinkage can occur as a result of the subserosal fibroids dying. Also, just as with UAE, success and failure of this procedure can be tracked by two different standards: **technical failure** and **clinical failure.** In addition, **complications** can occur during the procedure that result in injury, a less-than-desired outcome, or unanticipated results.

Technical Failure **Technical failures** are primarily related to the following:

1. skill of laparoscopic surgeon
2. location of the subserosal fibroid
3. size of the fibroid (a fibroid uterus greater than 10 cm is unlikely to have a successful outcome)

4. any number of additional odd circumstances that present themselves during the procedure.

Clinical Failure Clinical failure rates for myolysis generally involve failure of the fibroids to shrink significantly and continued problems with abnormal bleeding. Since myolysis and cryomyolysis only treat subserosal fibroids, many women may continue to have abnormal bleeding—particularly if an intramural fibroid moves to the submucosal region or a submucosal fibroid develops. In these cases, myolysis and cryomyolysis are not considered adequate procedures to effectively treat the fibroid-laden uterus alone. Often a secondary procedure must be performed to alleviate symptoms from additional fibroids other than those that are subserosal.

Unfortunately, there is limited research indicating how often additional fibroid symptoms occur. Research does indicate, however, that by only treating the subserosal fibroid through myolysis or cryomyolysis, recurrent fibroids causing additional problems are a very strong possibility. As a result, many women end up undergoing hysterectomy within five years of undergoing this procedure.

Dr. Herbert Goldfarb found that by combining myolysis with endometrial ablation or hysteroscopic resection (myomectomy) he was able to reduce the subsequent hysterectomy rate tremendously. Combining myolysis with endometrial ablation resulted in only 5.7 percent of women going on to a hysterectomy (within five years). Combining myolysis with hysteroscopic resection of submucosal fibroids reduced the hysterectomy rate to 3.5 percent (also within five years).

Complications Long-range studies showing complication rates for myolysis and cryomyolysis have not been published to date. Items that are considered potential risks are:

1. **Blood Transfusion.** If a severe blood loss occurs during either of these procedures or as a postoperative complication of these procedures, a blood transfusion may be necessary. In addition, an exploratory laparotomy (abdominal incision) may be necessary to repair a damaged blood vessel.
2. **Damage to Internal Organs.** With the use of laparoscopy, accidental injury to internal organs can occur. This might be the result of a per-

foration or a laceration by an instrument, or an electrosurgical burn may cause it. Further surgery may be necessary to repair the organ. This can occur at the time of the procedure or days/weeks after the surgery.

3. **Adhesion Formation.** After any pelvic or abdominal surgery, scar tissue (adhesions) can form. This may result in abdominal or pelvic pain, or intestinal obstruction. Further surgery may be necessary to remove the adhesions.

4. **Postoperative Infections.** Infection may develop at the site of surgery or at distant sites that may require antibiotics. It may also result in additional surgery. Severe infections after laparoscopic surgery are uncommon.

5. **Hernia.** A hernia (rupture) in the abdominal wall may occur, requiring further surgery.

6. **Side Effects of Lupron.** Common side effects include: cessation of your menstrual period, hot flashes, failure to shrink the fibroids, a possible worsening of your fibroids, skin reaction to the injection site, headaches, irregular vaginal bleeding, and vaginal dryness. The most critical side effect of Lupron, however, is the possibility of *irreversible* bone loss—osteoporosis—particularly if it is taken for more than six months.

Fertility and Myolysis

There appears to be conflicting information on the issue of fertility after myolysis. Some doctors say that myolysis is a good alternative to hysterectomy—especially for women who want to retain their ability to have children.

Others, such as Dr. William Parker, author of *A Gynecologist's Second Opinion: The Questions and Answers You Need to Take Charge of Your Health*, believes it is not a good alternative for women wishing to preserve their fertility. He indicates that neither myolysis nor cryomyolysis is recommended for women who still want to give birth to children and cites two major problems with the procedure:

1. Scar tissue (adhesions) has been known to form around the uterus after myolysis.

2. The strength of the uterine wall after myolysis is unknown.

Because of the potential risk of the uterus tearing during labor, it's important that women not attempt to get pregnant after myolysis or cryomyolysis, according to Dr. Parker.

Dr. Goldfarb, the physician who initiated this procedure in the United States, strongly agrees with Dr. Parker's assessment. In fact, he indicates that he has always been diligent about not offering this procedure to women who intend to become pregnant in the future. The risk of uterine rupture is simply too great. When a woman becomes pregnant after myolysis, she stands the risk of losing both her uterus *and* her baby. Nonetheless, some gynecologists offering this procedure have not shown due diligence in this regard, and several women have experienced uterine rupture with pregnancy as a result.

If you wish to retain your uterus for future childbearing, examine your options very closely before choosing myolysis or cryomyolysis as a treatment option!

History of Myolysis

Myolysis is a procedure that has been around since the late 1980s in Europe and was initially used as an alternative to myomectomy for women with fibroids who wanted to keep their uterus for future childbearing. Fertility rates turned out to be quite low, however, and pelvic adhesions were common. Needless to say, this procedure was quickly abandoned.

In the United States, not too many doctors perform myolysis. It's the "baby" of Dr. Goldfarb, as he introduced it to the U.S. gynecological community in 1990. It's unknown how many of these procedures have been performed in the United States to date, as the information has not been actively collected. However, Dr. Goldfarb did communicate to me that he performs around one hundred of these procedures annually.

Generally, most gynecologists don't know much about myolysis or cryomyolysis. In fact, only doctors who are thoroughly experienced laparoscopic operators should even attempt this procedure. Unless your gynecologist is a specialist in endoscopy, or open to referring you to another physician, you most likely will not be told about this procedure by your gynecologist or will be told that it is not an option for you. Well, maybe it is and maybe it isn't. You can begin to find out by asking your gynecologist questions about his skill with laparoscopic procedures.

Both skill and special equipment are required to perform this procedure, and this may well account for the low number of patients who have actually undergone this procedure. For more information or to locate a physician certified in endoscopy, be sure and check the Accreditation Council for Gynecologic Endoscopy (see chapter 8 for more information on this organization).

Hysterectomy

With hysterectomy, the uterus and all uterine fibroids are removed together. While the fibroids are eliminated, it is a bit like selling your house to get rid of uninvited relatives that won't go home, isn't it?

It all certainly sounds simple enough. You just check yourself in, get a surgeon to remove it all, and before you know it—there's nothing much left to write home about.

I wish it truly were that simple. Unfortunately, it is a surgical procedure filled with complications and poor outcomes for a very high percentage of women. Eleven in 10,000 women will die from this procedure and approximately another 30 percent will endure some sort of complications. In addition, many women are directed by their gynecologists to also have their cervix and ovaries removed during their hysterectomy for the prevention of cancer. Not for the actual presence of cancer. For the *prevention* of cancer. This, in turn, adds to the long list of complications and ongoing problems many women encounter after their hysterectomies.

Even with all the known complications of hysterectomy, it remains the number-one suggested and performed procedure for the treatment of uterine fibroids. Several hundred thousand women annually undergo hysterectomy for the treatment of their benign uterine fibroids and along with that, 60 percent choose to have their ovaries removed. Considering that a woman has less than 1.8 percent risk of being diagnosed with ovarian cancer in her lifetime, this 60 percent figure of ovary removal (oophorectomy) during hysterectomy is truly questionable. Particularly since it causes instant surgical menopause.

Without ovaries, hormone replacement therapy is a definite necessity. If a woman who no longer has ovaries chooses to disregard hormone replacement therapy or *is not directed to take hormone therapy by her gynecologist,* she is most certainly at increased risk for developing heart disease and osteoporosis. Heart disease just happens to be the number-one killer of women in America.

Ovarian Cancer

Women with a strong, clearly documented risk of ovarian cancer within their family may have a sound reason to perhaps ask the gynecological surgeon to remove their ovaries while performing their hysterectomy *even when they are not diseased or cancerous at all.* Around 7 percent of all ovarian cancer is thought to be genetically related. Women who have witnessed the painful death of a close family member to ovarian cancer would, therefore, have compelling reason to want to avoid that prospect for themselves. You should be aware, however, that an ovarian-type cancer could still occur in the pelvic region even without the presence of the ovaries—if you're destined to get this type of cancer, removing the ovaries does not, necessarily, protect you.

In addition to oophorectomy, the majority of women also have the cervix removed. If a woman has a history of cervical dysplasia, she may be at higher risk for cervical cancer and may definitely want to consider having the cervix removed. Even so, considering that the lifetime risk for diagnosis of cervical cancer is only .7 percent, why are so many doctors eager to remove the cervix from *all* women who undergo hysterectomy? After all, removing the cervix places a woman at an extremely high risk for post-hysterectomy complications that include urinary stress incontinence, prolapse, and sexual dysfunction.

Even with all the information provided in this book that clearly maps out the wide variety of alternative treatment options, let's say you're actually thinking about that hysterectomy the doctor insists is the only solution to your uterine fibroids. It sounds so curative and final. You find yourself dreaming about taking those fibroids and the mess they keep making around "your house" and actually moving them out forever. No more bleeding and no more worrying about pain or bulk symptoms. Ah, geez. It sounds so wonderful. But then you mention to your friends and family that you're thinking about a hysterectomy, and they immediately flip on the light switch and start giving you the third degree—asking all kinds of questions—and you don't have the answers. Questions like:

- What kind of hysterectomy? (*What? There's more than one kind of hysterectomy? My doctor never mentioned that . . .)*
- Are you keeping your cervix and ovaries? (*I don't know. The doctor said they should come out so I don't have to ever worry about cancer.)*
- Will you need to take hormones (*Huh? The doctor never said **anything** about* that!)

The questions are endless, and you probably don't have the answers. But these first three questions should be a clue to you that there is potential for a lot of research and work to be done both before and after you undergo this procedure. It may seem that OTHER people have more questions of you (and your doctor) than YOU even thought of, and you're beginning to wonder just which layer of the ozone your brain has been floating around in!

Women you know start throwing acronyms at you . . . better find out what your FSH is before the procedure so you can better gauge your HRT afterwards . . . By the way, are you having a SH, LSH, LAH, LAVH, TAH, or TAH/BSO? *Say what?!* Get out that pencil and pad and start taking note of all of the questions you encounter because you're probably going to need to return to your doctor and talk a bit more about this procedure he's recommended.

In the meantime, welcome. You've just joined **The Club.** All women who've been given the *"You need a hysterectomy"* statement by their doctor will know *EXACTLY* what I mean—and you will, too, before much longer. This elite group of women numbers in the millions, and all of us know that most women don't even think about us or the possibility of hysterectomy. Until, that is, they too receive the *"You need a hysterectomy"* statement from their doctor.

Speaking for the entire group of women who have joined **The Club,** I can tell you that we want to help you the best way we can with whatever collective experiences we can share. Right now, I feel confident in saying that **The Club's** collective experiences tell us the following:

*If you are a woman suffering from **ONLY** uterine fibroids, you may very well **NOT** need a hysterectomy.*

Please turn around, go back through that door, and talk to your doctor some more. You need more answers. You need to be asking the questions that could, very well, allow you to keep your uterus, cervix, and ovaries intact. Believe me when I say, *You can find a better way to get rid of the relatives and keep the house if you really try!*

There are less drastic treatment options for taking care of your bleeding, pain, and bulk symptoms. I hope you will turn to hysterectomy as only a last resort when all else fails. *Every homeless person in America will tell you without a doubt that once you lose your home and have nothing to replace it with, it's really, really hard to get back on your feet again and move forward. It can be done. But it's not easy, and some do not succeed. The same can be said for hysterectomy.*

There is simply no turning back from this *potential* roller-coaster ride of complications and hormonal deprivation. If you can avoid it, please do.

Don't You Have Anything GOOD to Say about Hysterectomy?

Yes. I do. Even though I wouldn't recommend this treatment option for benign uterine fibroids, it is important to remember that many women find hysterectomy an absolute lifesaver—particularly **when all other treatment options fail to resolve their symptoms** or **because of cancer**. In addition, as many as 70 percent of all women who undergo hysterectomy report satisfaction in their procedure choice and treatment outcome. A common statement voiced by these women is:

"My only regret is that I didn't have it done sooner."
—Cheri

Clearly, the *majority* of women undergoing hysterectomy report a positive outcome. On the other hand, what about the incredibly high number of women that make up the *minority* who are dissatisfied due to complications or poor outcome?

"I'll never be able to live a normal life again. I'm in constant pain, depressed, and barely able to function. The doctor who did this to me seems to think it's all in my head and has prescribed antidepressants. Now what do I do? I'm much worse off than I was before the surgery and totally lost on how to fix this. It seems that all I've done is trade one set of symptoms for another. It's been five years now and I'm tired of being sick all of the time. I just want my life back."
—Joan

It's a very serious decision to make; undergoing a hysterectomy can, and often does, change the quality of your life forever. Sometimes for the better. Sometimes for the worse. Sometimes, we simply don't have a choice in the matter. Roughly 10 percent of all hysterectomies are performed to stop the spread of cancer—so we do know that hysterectomy can save lives.

Uterine fibroids, however, are *not* cancerous. They can be life threatening, though, if they are not treated in a timely and appropriate fashion.

This section will do its best to give you the information you need to make an informed decision about hysterectomy.

Hysterectomy Procedures

There are six variations on a theme when it comes to hysterectomy. Well, there are actually more than six, but this section covers the primary choices normally presented to women with uterine fibroids.

1. laparoscopic supracervical hysterectomy (LSH)
2. (abdominal) supracervical hysterectomy (SH)
3. laparoscopic assisted vaginal hysterectomy (LAVH)
4. total vaginal hysterectomy (TVH)
5. total abdominal hysterectomy (TAH)
6. total abdominal hysterectomy/bilateral salpingo oophorectomy (TAH/BSO)

The most important differences among these types of hysterectomies have to do with whether or not the cervix and ovaries are removed along with the uterus. A *supracervical* hysterectomy is also referred to as a *subtotal* hysterectomy and refers to the removal of only the uterus. "Supra" means *above* and, in this case, placed with the word *cervical* it means "above the cervix." LSH and SH are both supracervical and subtotal hysterectomies allowing you to retain your cervix.

Each of the four remaining types of hysterectomy in the above list is considered *total* hysterectomy where both the uterus and cervix are removed. In addition to that, with TAH/BSO, the fallopian tubes (salpingo) and ovaries (oophor) are also removed.

Since the laparoscope allows for a smaller incision (generally through the navel) and access to your reproductive organs, the uterus, cervix (for LAVH), and all your fibroids must be chopped up (morcellated) in order to be suctioned out. If your fibroid uterus is too large for this, you may be asked to undergo Lupron injections as a pretreatment to shrink your fibroids.

While abdominal incisions for hysterectomy were, once upon a time, the mainstay of all hysterectomies for a fibroid uterus, it is now deemed unnecessary the vast majority of the time. Only extreme cases of particularly huge fibroids truly require an abdominal incision today. Even so, the vast majority of hysterectomies performed today are still total abdominal hysterectomies.

With an abdominal approach, an incision is made either horizontally across the top of your pubic hairline or vertically between the navel and the top of your pubic hairline. Horizontal incisions heal quicker and are preferred by just about everyone. I honestly can't imagine why some doctors still perform the vertical incision, but they do. Rumor has it that some surgeons tell patients that their size of fibroid uterus *requires* a vertical incision. Nonsense. It is highly unlikely that any fibroid uterus would require a vertical incision. Vertical incisions run perpendicular to the natural lines of the skin, and overweight people often have serious problems with healing when their skin is constantly tugging against this type of incision. In an effort to help his overweight patients avoid complications from the surgical incision, Dr. Hermann Johannn Pfannensteil came up with the horizontal incision. (Indeed, the horizontal incision was named Pfannensteil to honor this surgeon for this advancement in surgical technique.)

If you're still uncertain regarding the need for a vertical versus horizontal incision, consider this: C-sections are quite regularly performed with a horizontal incision. If a surgeon can remove a full-term baby out of this type of incision, it certainly makes sense that an extremely large fibroid uterus would also fit through it. It truly is important to discuss the type of incision your surgeon will be making in advance of the surgery so that you can obtain a better understanding of what he intends to do and why.

Vaginal hysterectomies are also frequently recommended to women who wish to avoid an abdominal incision. In fact, 25 percent of all hysterectomies are vaginal. Because all cutting and removing of the uterus and cervix occurs through the vagina, you will not have an abdominal incision to recover from or a resulting scar. This generally speeds up the recovery process as well. It may, however, have an impact on critical nerves in the vaginal region that results in reduced or complete lack of feelings during sex. So, the trade-off for that scar and recovery time *may* be an increased risk of sexual dysfunction.

There are several conditions that make vaginal hysterectomies more difficult—a history of prior pelvic surgery with the possible development of adhesions and/or the presence of endometriosis. As with a laparoscopic hysterectomy, if your fibroid uterus is too large for vaginal removal, you may be asked to undergo Lupron injections or some other form of GnRH as a pretreatment to shrink your fibroids.

There does seem to be some debate over the relative merits of vaginal hysterectomy versus abdominal hysterectomy. In the end, only you can decide which of the considerations brought to the debate are truly important.

Laparoscopic Supracervical Hysterectomy (LSH) Through use of a laparoscope, this type of hysterectomy removes the uterus but leaves your cervix in place. Leaving the cervix in place is said to cause less trauma as it leaves the pelvic "floor" intact. This helps to stop or reduce the chances of pelvic prolapse (the dropping or protrusion of organs into the vagina) or urinary stress incontinence at a later time. In addition, leaving the cervix in place allows the full length of the vagina to be fully preserved. Since your fibroid uterus is chopped up and suctioned out through the laparoscope, there is no abdominal incision to recover from, less discomfort and pain, and a relatively quick recovery time. This procedure is typically performed on an outpatient basis and you are generally released from the hospital within eighteen hours. Barring any complications, you should be back to normal activities within a week or so.

(Abdominal) Supracervical Hysterectomy (SH) Through an abdominal incision, this type of hysterectomy removes the uterus but leaves your cervix in place. With an extremely large fibroid uterus, an abdominal incision may be required in order for the surgeon to safely handle your internal organs and remove the fibroids and uterus. The hospital stay for an abdominal hysterectomy is three to five days with a recovery period of six to eight weeks.

Laparoscopic-Assisted Vaginal Hysterectomy (LAVH) Whenever endometriosis is also present with uterine fibroids, a LAVH is the preferred method of hysterectomy. Endometriosis located throughout the pelvic region can be removed along with the uterus with the use of the laparoscope. The laparoscope is used first to visualize the endometriosis and remove it, and then the uterus and cervix are removed vaginally.

Any time the cervix is removed along with the uterus, a number of additional complications may occur. These include:

1. shortening of the vagina
2. weakening of the support ligaments of the vagina
3. perforation of the bowels or critical blood vessels

In order to remove the cervix, the cardinal and utero-sacral ligaments that support your pelvic organs and hold them in place are cut. The cervix is removed and the whole thing is stitched up with the creation of a vaginal cuff. *(Much like a shirtsleeve that's been folded up and cuffed only in this case it's stitched in place.)* As you can imagine, this cutting of the ligaments does weaken the support structure that you were born with, and the creation of the cuff shortens the overall length of the vagina just as it does when you cuff a shirtsleeve. Both of these situations can lead to serious complications when the cervix is removed.

Total Vaginal Hysterectomy (TVH) With TVH, your fibroid uterus and cervix are removed completely through the vagina. Again, your fibroid uterus must be small enough to fit through the vaginal canal.

Total Abdominal Hysterectomy (TAH) With TAH, your fibroid uterus and cervix are removed through an abdominal incision.

Total Abdominal Hysterectomy with Bilateral Salpingo Oophorectomy (TAH/BSO) With TAH/BSO, your uterus, cervix, fallopian tubes, and ovaries are all removed abdominally. Some women and doctors refer to TAH/BSO as a "total pelvic clean out." Even so, because of cancer or advanced endometriosis or other disease of the pelvic region *in addition to uterine fibroids,* this procedure has been known to both improve and save the lives of women.

Ideal Hysterectomy Patient

The American College of Obstetricians and Gynecologists (ACOG) has identified the following guidelines for determining the ideal patient for the recommendation of hysterectomy when uterine fibroids are present. Using these guidelines, gynecologists can choose to remove your uterus during the performance of any pelvic surgery if any one or more of the following are present.

1. asymptomatic fibroids of a size that can be felt abdominally and are a concern to the patient
2. excessive uterine bleeding as shown by either of the following:
    ➤ excessive bleeding with flooding or clots or repeated menstrual periods lasting more than eight days
    ➤ anemia due to acute or chronic blood loss
3. pelvic discomfort fitting any one of the following categories:
    ➤ acute and severe
    ➤ chronic lower-abdominal or low-back pressure
    ➤ bladder pressure with urinary frequency not due to a urinary tract infection

The following are the ACOG guidelines for determining when **NOT** to recommend hysterectomy for uterine fibroids:

1. a woman's desire to maintain fertility (in this case, myomectomy should be discussed)
2. asymptomatic fibroids that are less than twelve weeks pregnancy in size.

About Those ACOG Guidelines . . .

Even if you wish to retain your uterus and do not want a hysterectomy, the ACOG guidelines protect gynecologists from legal recourse should they choose to perform a hysterectomy anyway while surgically treating your fibroids. If, for example, you are undergoing a myomectomy, you must put it in **writing** that you do **not** want a hysterectomy under any circumstances other than those necessary to save your life. Specific instructions to the physician should be noted on the hospital admitting forms as well as the informed consent document for surgery.

Successes, Failures, and Complications Where uterine fibroids are concerned, hysterectomy is considered to be the most successful, definitive cure that exists. When you remove the uterus along with all your fibroids, it's not likely that your fibroids will grow back! This is the ultimate success that can be had for the treatment of uterine fibroids.

In terms of failure, if you are having a hysterectomy because of abnormal bleeding, you need to know that even with the removal of your uterus abnormal bleeding is still a possibility. It seems odd; considering your uterus (and, consequently the endometrium) is removed with this procedure that you would still have bleeding. But, some women do. Typically, it is light and not excessive at all: more a surprise than a real nuisance to most women to whom this occurs.

Complications and complication rates vary depending upon the type of hysterectomy performed. In addition to the risk of death (about 11 per 10,000), the following are considered potential risks of hysterectomy:

1. **Blood Transfusion.** If a severe blood loss occurs during or after the procedure, a blood transfusion may be necessary. This occurs approximately 10 percent of the time. In addition, an exploratory laparotomy (abdominal incision) may be necessary to repair a damaged blood vessel.
2. **Damage to Internal Organs.** Accidental injury to internal organs can occur with any form of hysterectomy. This might be the result of a perforation or a laceration by an instrument, or an electrosurgical

burn may cause it. Further surgery may be necessary to repair the organ. This can occur at the time of the procedure or days/weeks after the surgery. Reoperation to investigate uncontrolled hemorrhage or to repair bladder, bowel, or ureteral injuries is necessary a little less than 1 percent of the time. In addition, up to 3 percent of women will develop some form of urinary complications other than infection.

3. **Adhesion Formation.** After any pelvic or abdominal surgery, scar tissue (adhesions) can form. This may result in abdominal or pelvic pain, or intestinal obstruction. Up to 2 percent may need additional surgery to remove adhesions from the bowel.

4. **Postoperative.** Infection may develop at the site of surgery or at distant sites that may require antibiotics. It may also result in additional surgery. Improper healing, narrowing of the vagina, and a heavy discharge are additional postoperative complications. Severe infections after laparoscopic surgery are uncommon.

5. **Hernia.** A hernia (rupture) in the abdominal wall may occur. If so, this would require further surgery.

6. **Ureter Damage.** Up to 1 percent may be damaged due to laceration, inadvertent binding of the ureter (ligation), compression, or puncture. This happens more often with abdominal hysterectomies than with vaginal hysterectomies. Reoperation may be required to repair ureter damage.

7. **Vaginal Vault Prolapse.** If not secured properly when the uterus is removed, the vagina will prolapse—that is, fall right on down and out.

8. **Blood Clots.** Rare but potentially deadly. Typically form in the legs but can travel to the lungs or brain.

9. **Prolapse of the Fallopian Tube.** Rare. Results in watery discharge, postcoital spotting, or abdominal/pelvic pain.

10. **Residual Ovarian Syndrome.** Pelvic pain and a possible development of a mass when the ovaries were retained.

11. **Menopause.** Women who have their ovaries removed experience surgical menopause. Even when ovaries are NOT removed, 20 percent of the remaining group of women undergoing hysterectomy experience premature menopause.

12. **Sexual Dysfunction.** Around 20 percent of women experience a negative impact on sexual function post-hysterectomy. The number of women who experience sexual dysfunction when oophorectomy is performed with hysterectomy may be as high as 46 percent.

Is That It?

No. I wish it were. Please don't forget that permanently removing an organ from your body is major surgery. This list of complications was not put together to scare you—merely to inform you of the possibilities. Some of the above-listed complications are extremely rare—but they have occurred or they wouldn't be on the list.

In reality, the three most common complications of hysterectomy are fever, urinary tract infection, and wound infection. Fever, as a complication, is generally indicative of either a urinary tract infection and/or a wound infection, and 15 percent of all hysterectomy patients will experience a fever at or above 100.5°. Because of the use of a Foley catheter to collect urine during a hysterectomy, urinary tract infections will affect as many as 10 percent of all patients. "Other" infections pop up about 10 percent of the time and include: vaginal cuff abscess, pelvic abscess, blood poisoning, pneumonia, and an inflammation of any number of the different layers of your abdominal wall.

A Word About Heart Disease

Heart disease is the number-one killer of women in the United States. Every year over 350,000 women die of coronary disease in this country and there has now been, unfortunately, a very clear link established to both natural and surgical menopause to this statistic. With the decline of estrogen in the body as a result of menopause, a woman's "bad" cholesterol (LDL—low-density lipoprotein) levels rise and begin building up fat in the coronary arteries. This may well contribute to what we know is an overall increased incidence of heart disease in menopausal women. Some numbers to think about:

- ~600,000 hysterectomies are performed each year in this country.
- ~50% of all hysterectomies are performed on women who are under the age of 40.
- ~66% of all hysterectomies are performed on women in their thirties and forties.
- ~60% of women undergoing hysterectomy choose to have their ovaries removed and therefore place themselves into immediate surgical menopause.

- ~20% of the remaining 40% of women who retain their ovaries with hysterectomy experience premature ovarian failure.

With the decline of estrogen now being directly tied to coronary disease in women, is it any wonder at all with numbers like these that heart disease is the number-one killer of women in America today? Thinking about this, two more questions cross my mind. Over 37 percent of all women in American will undergo a hysterectomy by the age of sixty. What I want to know is:

1. What percentage of the women who die each year as a result of heart disease underwent hysterectomy at some point in their lifetime?
2. Is that statistic higher or lower than for the portion of the female population who did NOT choose to undergo hysterectomy?

A Word About Psychological Stressors

Oh, the studies that have been done. Okay, here's what we "sort of" know:

- *Depression is a major complication of hysterectomy.*
- Depression *before* hysterectomy is a solid indicator that there will be depression *after* hysterectomy.
- The shorter the amount of time between making a decision to undergo hysterectomy and the actual procedure, the greater the chance of depression.
- Estrogen stimulates the release of endorphins (*"pain numbing" proteins in the brain*) from the hypothalamus. But 60 percent of women who undergo hysterectomy have their ovaries removed . . . no more estrogen . . . so much for the release of endorphins.

Now for the controversy. Is depression after a hysterectomy psychological or physiological? Or, both? Is it all in your mind or do disrupted hormones play a part? And how about that long list of complications—what role does suffering from complications post-hysterectomy play in depression? If I had a urinary tract infection that took forever to go away or perhaps had to undergo a secondary operation to repair something from my hysterectomy, would I be depressed? Yes, I think so.

How about the loss of sexual arousal or function? Ovaries manufacture testosterone while the vagina, cervix, and uterus play a role in sending signals to the central nervous system of your brain that allows you to feel pleasure and orgasm with sex. Without ovaries and with surgical alterations in the vagina, cervix, and uterus, isn't it possible that these physical changes might suddenly present problems resulting in depression?

I could write questions about this issue all night and still not resolve a thing. There is a gap between what doctors verbalize to patients about hysterectomy and depression and the truth. A huge gap. Research has not bridged that gap. Why not? Because the majority of researchers thus far were not interested in looking at physiological reasons behind depression. To do so would point to a *problem with the hysterectomy* instead of a problem with the patient's mental state and predisposition toward depression. Poorly put together questionnaires predetermine the outcome of many a study.

My suggestion to doctors involved in hysterectomy research? The next time you do a study on this issue and need to put together a questionnaire, please consider involving women who've *experienced* hysterectomy and depression. Involve patient advocates who've sat in on support groups and helped women who've *experienced* this side effect of hysterectomy. In short, perhaps it would be a good idea to combine your *medical knowledge and experience* with the *practical and personal experiences* of women who've undergone hysterectomy. These women have solid information to share with you and can help to validate your research plan, if you let them.

History of Hysterectomy

The first reported case of an abdominal hysterectomy was performed in Manchester, England, in 1843. It was an abdominal supracervical hysterectomy (SH) for a fibroid uterus. The woman died two weeks later. It wasn't a great beginning.

The first *successful* (that is, the woman actually survived) hysterectomy was not performed for ten more years—in 1853. It was performed by Dr. Ellis Burnham in Massachusetts and, like that very first case, was also supracervical. In fact, all the early hysterectomies performed were supracervical as this allowed physicians to avoid entering what they considered the *contaminated* area of the vagina. In addition to that, they deliberately avoided removing the cervix because of the increased bleeding they encountered when attempting to do so. Of course, there were no antibiotics in 1853 to deal with infections, and blood transfusions were unheard of for treating blood loss during surgical procedures. Furthermore, all procedures at that time were performed without anesthetics. Is it any wonder that 70 to 90 percent of hysterectomy patients died?

The first total abdominal hysterectomy (TAH) in the United States was performed by Dr. Edward Richardson at Johns Hopkins University 1929. In performing this procedure, he chose to remove both the uterus and the cervix. The cervix was not removed to treat cervical cancer, but to simply *prevent* cervical cancer from occurring. This was the single procedure that set the pace for all future total abdominal hysterectomies in the United States.

The first successful vaginal hysterectomy (VH) was performed for cancer of the cervix in 1824 by Dr. Recamier.

Although successful techniques for both abdominal and vaginal hysterectomy were clearly developed by 1900, physicians have continued to debate which approach is best for the last 100 years. From 1900 through the 1940s, subtotal hysterectomy was performed most often in the United States. It was considered simpler, safer, and had fewer risks of complications and lower blood loss compared to total abdominal hysterectomy. During the 1940s and 1950s, there was tremendous debate on a national level over the issue of removing the cervix during a hysterectomy as a *preventive* measure against cancer. Apparently, that debate has remained unresolved as the practice of prophylactically removing the cervix during hysterectomy continues quite heartily today and ongoing studies looking at risks and benefits of doing so are still actively occurring.

The introduction of laparoscopic assisted vaginal hysterectomy (LAVH) by Dr. Harry Reich was the first real change in a very long time in the world of hysterectomy. In 1976, while using laparoscopic equipment, Dr. Harry Reich pioneered a new way to do hysterectomy that does not require a lengthy abdominal incision and allows the patient to recover more quickly than ever before. Although this technique was developed in 1976, it did not become widely recognized by gynecologists until the medical paper titled "Laparoscopic Hysterectomy" was published in the *Journal of Gynecological Surgery* in 1989. It took thirteen years for this procedure to be recognized in the medical community as a viable treatment option, but even today many insurance providers still consider laparoscopic surgery "investigational."

Of course, it wasn't long before someone chose to come along and one-up Dr. Reich with a laparoscopic *supracervical* hysterectomy (LSH). With research out of Finland showing better sexual function if the cervix is left intact, Dr. Thomas Lyons set out to do just that when he came up with laparoscopic supracervical hysterectomy in 1990. Thanks to this new technique (and the study out of Finland), between 1991 and 1996 the number of supracervical hysterectomies being performed in the United States increased by 250 percent!

During the last 150 years or so of hysterectomy procedures and slow but sure technical advances, doctors have gone back and forth between recommending supracervical hysterectomy or the total removal of uterus and cervix with a total hysterectomy. It's interesting to note that in most medical literature doctors write about the *decisions women make* to either keep or remove their cervix as though different generations of women go back and forth on this issue all on their own. It seems so perplexing to these doctors. In one decade supracervical is "popular" and then in the very next decade it's out of vogue and total hysterectomy is "in." Then, *violà!* a new technique is devised and supracervical is back in again. *Hmmmm.* Do doctors truly not understand that women make decisions about medical procedures based on the information presented to them by their physicians? Do doctors also not understand that choices made by women are directly related to the choices created and presented to those very women by their physician? Certainly the doctors who are out there perfecting their techniques and trying new ways to do things are "sharing" their information with their patients in a way that influences the decisions that are made. Wouldn't you think?

New advances in medicine are always welcome. Perfecting old procedures and turning them into something less invasive, less prone to complications, and of greater benefit to a patient's overall recovery process is wonderful. Truly. I just wish doctors would stop writing about the "choices women make" as though they really made them *completely of their own accord.* Not a single medical procedure would be performed on this planet if a doctor weren't there to recommend it.

At any rate, if you find that you truly *do* need a hysterectomy or you simply choose—for whatever personal reason—to go ahead with a hysterectomy, it is my hope that the information in this section helped to answer some of your questions about the procedure. To learn about each type of hysterectomy procedure in greater depth and based upon your specific circumstances, I would urge you to write out all your questions on paper and then schedule an extra-long appointment with your gynecologist to discuss the details and get answers.

Another way to gather information and get answers is to join one of the many support groups that are available on the Internet or in your community. They can prove instrumental in helping you through your hysterectomy, as many women who have lived through exactly what you're about to go through are in those support groups waiting with open arms to help you. Join **before** you have the procedure, if you can, because the support you need begins **now.**

Hysterectomy Support

One of the best hysterectomy support groups on the Internet today is Sans Uteri. This group was founded by Beth Tiner of **Findings: The Women's Healthcare Advocacy Service** in 1996.

All email posted to this group is moderated by Beth and placed into a single email, digestlike format and sent out only once each day. Those considering hysterectomy as well as those who've had a hysterectomy are welcome to join. This is a strong, well-founded, sharing support group.

To subscribe, send a blank email message to:
SANS-UTERI@FINDINGS.NET
Type the word **SUBSCRIBE** in the subject line of your email.
   website:www.findings.net/sans-uteri.html

Stacking the Deck?

At this point in the chapter, you're probably wondering why anybody would *choose* a hysterectomy for the treatment of her benign uterine fibroids when it is filled with the potential for so much negative outcome. It may well look as though I've stacked the deck of cards pretty heavily against hysterectomy. If so, it truly wasn't intentional. This procedure is a definite lifesaver for women with cancerous disease of the uterus. Hysterectomy is, however, a procedure that is simply filled with the potential for problems. The items in this chapter did not come out of my overactive imagination. They are real, and patients and physicians alike have reported them.

When it comes to benign uterine fibroids, some women simply don't like the idea of a tumor, dead or alive, remaining in their bodies. They don't want to go through myomectomy only to have to do it again if new fibroids grow, and merely "shrinking" the fibroids and leaving bulky dead tissue in their bodies is unacceptable to them. Others are afraid of cancer. Very. Even small statistics like a 1.8 percent chance of ovarian cancer or a .7 percent chance of cervical cancer in their lifetime seems frightening.

Some women just don't want to be bothered with the details. Comments like "I just want to do it and get it over with so I can get on with my life" are not unusual from these women. Unfortunately, since the complication rate is rather high with hysterectomy, a great many of these women wander back into support groups six months or a year later very upset that complications happened to *them*. They thought positive thoughts, expected a good outcome, and now are struggling with aftereffects of the surgery.

But there are women who've had tremendous success with hysterectomy. There are a lot of them. If, over the last twenty years, 12 million hysterectomies have been performed and 70 percent of them were relatively complication-free, that makes for about 8,400,000 women walking around who didn't have a negative surgical experience. Of course, that also means that roughly 3,600,000 did have a negative experience. Only you can weigh the risks and benefits and decide whether or not hysterectomy is the right thing to do for your specific circumstances.

Additional Treatment Options

The treatment options covered in this section are separated out for good reason: each one comes with enough limitations to warrant special discussion. Clinical research, Lupron, mifepristone, and female reconstructive surgery (FRS) are all certainly options for fibroid treatment. While clinical research is a critical and necessary part of making advances in medicine, it does require more diligence on the part of the participant to truly know and understand the research if she is to appropriately protect herself. Each of the remaining three options presented here has an interesting and controversial history that deserves a closer look.

Clinical Research

With every passing week, more and more researchers are joining the current scientific community that is working on finding a "cure" for uterine fibroids. Around the world, researchers are looking for new drug therapies, refining current procedures, and developing new procedures altogether—to help women suffering from uterine fibroids. Unfortunately, the research may be too far off to help those of us who have fibroids *today*.

On the other hand, there are quite a few clinical trials that involve a variety of *potential* solutions. Because researchers seem to be turning up the heat on finding cures or better treatments, more and more clinical trials are started every day. If you are certain that none of the treatment solutions outlined in this chapter fits your needs, rest assured that it may be only a matter of time before new solutions rise out of the current clinical research. If you don't want to wait for the outcome of these trials (*or you CAN'T wait for the outcome of the trials!*), you can always take the necessary steps to join one. Someone has to participate and contribute to the body of knowledge that we have on uterine fibroids. Maybe that someone is you. Consider this: Ongoing research in the area of uterine fibroids will help *millions* of women who will, in the future, most certainly find themselves facing this disease.

The Agency for Health Care Policy and Research (AHCPR) is an arm of the United States Department of Health and Human Services and was created to pull together information about health care and the health-care system in the United States. This is a terrific place to begin looking for information on clinical trials, as this agency's mission is to "support, conduct, and disseminate research." Start with requesting a copy of the AHCPR publication, "What Are Clinical Trials All About" to begin learning more about how clinical trial research is carried out in the United States. For a complete listing of all AHCPR published documents, contact:

AHCPR Publications Clearinghouse
P. O. Box 8547
Silver Spring, MD 20907

1 (800) 358-9295 (toll-free in the United States)
(410) 381-3150 (outside the United States)
1 (888) 586-6340 (toll-free TDD)
http://www.ahcpr.gov

To find out how you can actually participate in ongoing research on uterine fibroids and treatment options, there are a couple of additional agencies you can contact. The first is the National Institute of Health (NIH). The NIH is an agency of the U.S. Department of Health and Human Services and is made up of twenty-five separate health institutes and centers. This agency receives nearly $16 billion dollars a year to conduct research and support research of nonfederal scientists in universities, medical schools, hospitals, and research institutions. Clinical trial information for these agencies can be found on the NIH website (http://www.nih.gov/health/).

CenterWatch, Inc., is a Boston-based publishing company that focuses and collects information on the clinical trials industry. Ongoing clinical trials are listed on their website, but information can also be obtained by contacting:

CenterWatch, Inc.
22 Thomson Place, 12F3
Boston, MA 02210-1212
1 (800) 765-9647
Email: cntrwatch@aol.com
http://www.centerwatch.com

Finally, according to the AHCPR, a clinical "study" is not quite the same thing as a clinical "trial." Many doctors do ask patients to participate in "studies" as a way to gather information on a specific treatment or drug (FDA approved drugs, that is), and the information collected is usually published. While this does add to the body of information that scientists have on a specific treatment or drug, it is simply not the same thing as a clinical trial at all. Clinical trials are much more tightly controlled research studies that are based on a protocol, or set of rules, that determines precisely who can participate, what tests, procedures, medications, etc., are given, and the length of the trial. There is usually no cost to the participant in a clinical trial. To ensure that strict guidelines and safeguards are followed and to protect the participants in a trial, all clinical trials are approved and monitored by an Institutional Review Board (IRB).

Advantages/Disadvantages of Participating in a Clinical Trial

Upside	Downside
Use of new medication and procedures well before they are available to the public	Unknown risks, side effects, long-term complications of medications and procedures
Free medications, diagnostic tests, procedures	Medications or procedures may be placebos
Close monitoring of your health	Following requirements and undergoing frequent monitoring may take a lot of time and effort
Access to physicians who may be the best in their area of medicine	Physicians may be influenced by money received from pharmaceuticals and device manufacturers and NOT performing a study in your best interest or reporting results accurately
Knowledge that you are contributing to science and society	Contributions to science and medicine won't help YOU if you receive placebos or experience side effects or complications

Lupron (Gonadotropin Releasing Hormones—GnRH)

Perimenopausal women are sometimes recommended the drug Lupron for the treatment of their uterine fibroids. Lupron is a gonadotropin releasing hormone (GnRH) antagonist usually given by injection on a monthly basis. This drug blocks the production of estrogen and puts you into a state of artificial (chemically induced) menopause. Since fibroids need estrogen to continue growing, Lupron helps to shrink the fibroids, just as they would if you were to suddenly enter natural menopause.

Lupron as a stand-alone medical treatment for uterine fibroids is filled with many drawbacks. For starters, it can't be used for more than three to six months at a time. Why not? Because severe, ongoing estrogen deprivation causes osteoporosis (severe bone loss and decreased bone density, which can result in fractures). In fact, Lupron is so effective as an estrogen blocker that it places the body into a state of **irreversible** osteoporosis if it is used for longer than six months at a time. On the other hand, the minute you discontinue using Lupron, the fibroids begin growing back. Within six months, they're back to the same size as they were previously—sometimes larger. Clearly this is a yo-yo treatment plan that doesn't really solve the problem of uterine fibroids at all.

Additional side effects from Lupron include:

- cessation of your menstrual period
- hot flashes
- a possible worsening of your fibroids
- skin reaction to the injection site
- headaches
- irregular vaginal bleeding
- vaginal dryness.

(The above list represents the side effects documented as part of the clinical trials research. They are not, however, the full picture.)

Some women swear by this drug. It helped get them "over the hump" and into menopause while stopping their excessive bleeding and shrinking their fibroids. For others, it was a way to shrink their fibroids and prepare them for an easier myomectomy or hysterectomy. In the following case, Betsy had Lupron injections for five months prior to a vaginal hysterectomy.

"Lupron has been a VERY POSITIVE experience for me . . . and with only seven weeks or so of mild hot flashes versus an extremely violent and overwhelming menstrual cycle . . . I am thrilled."

According to Betsy, without Lupron and the subsequent shrinkage of her fibroids, her hysterectomy would have been abdominal.

While many women have registered successful stories of their Lupron use with minimal side effects, others have horror stories to tell.

> *"It has been two years since my Lupron injections and I suffer from severe pain in the right leg (femoral neuropathy), sciatic nerve damage, arthritis in the lower back, diabetes—which was immediate after the second shot—and I now walk with a limp thanks to all of these side effects."*
> —Paula

There are many unsettling facts about this drug. To begin with, the Food and Drug Administration (FDA) has over ten thousand adverse reaction complaints registered against Lupron on file. And, while Lupron is an FDA approved drug, it has never been approved as a fibroid treatment or as a presurgical treatment for the shrinkage of fibroids. Using Lupron to shrink uterine fibroids is an off-label use of the drug. (*See chapter 3, The Choices.*)

Additionally, research reports on certain National Institutes of Health–funded clinical trials of Lupron for use with fibroids and endometriosis were discredited when principal investigator Dr. Andrew J. Friedman was found to have falsified and fabricated approximately 80 percent of the data in two reports published in the medical journals *Fertility and Sterility* ("Gonadotrophin-releasing hormone agonist plus estrogen-progestin 'add-back' therapy for endometriosis-related pelvic pain," 1993) and *Obstetrics and Gynecology* ("Does low-dose combination oral contraceptive use affect uterine size or menstrual flow in premenopausal women with leiomyomas?" 1995). Friedman also altered and fabricated information in permanent patient medical records in order to provide support for the reports. The discredited reports were ultimately retracted, but they are only two of more than fifty papers published by Friedman on related research that are presumably still relied on by doctors for treatment decisions today and into the future. In 1996 Dr. Friedman, formerly director of reproductive endocrinology at Brigham and Women's Hospital, entered into an agreement excluding him from U.S. government–supported research for three years, and in 1998 he was disciplined by the Massachusetts medical board, which suspended his medical license and fined him $10,000. The board allowed Friedman to petition for a stay of the suspension after a year, and its public records indicate that the suspension was stayed in 1999, meaning Friedman's medical license could be reinstated.

To report a suspected adverse side effect from Lupron (or any drug or medical device), call the Food and Drug Administration at (888) INFO-FDA. Medical consumers can also file reports on the Internet at http://www.fda.gov (click on MedWatch Medical Products Reporting). According to the FDA, a patient's identity is held in strict confidence by the FDA and protected to the fullest extent of the law. In addition, you may also contact the following for additional information on reporting side effects:

➤ TAP Pharmaceuticals Medical Services Department
   (800) 622-2011
   http://www.lupron.com
➤ The National Lupron Victims Network
   (609) 858-2131
   http://www.voicenet.com/~nlvn

So what use *is* Lupron approved for with women? In 1995, the FDA granted approval for Lupron use with the following limitations:

"Lupron depot 3.75 mg and iron therapy are indicated for the preoperative hematologic improvement of patients with anemia caused by uterine fibroids."

The FDA recommended a one-month trial period of iron first to stem the tide of anemia (confirmed with a hematocrit lower than 35) due to blood loss caused by fibroids and indicated that Lupron could be added if, after one month, iron was inadequate. The recommended amount of time for taking Lupron was three months. Information on the safety of this drug for periods of time longer than six months based on medical research is unknown. The FDA specifically recommended that this drug NOT be used for more than six months, not "six months at a time"; it was not recommended for use for more than six months *total* in the lifetime of a patient.

As you can read, there are a lot of good reasons why Lupron was not on my "top 10" list of medical treatments for uterine fibroids. Regardless of how many success stories there are—like Betsy's—the number of unanswered questions about this drug make me extremely nervous as a medical consumer. If you do choose to go with your doctor's recommendation on the use of Lupron, please be certain that your benefits outweigh the multitude of known risks.

Mifepristone

Mifepristone, formerly known as RU-486, is an interesting drug with an almost unbelievable political history. While it shows tremendous promise for the potential treatment of a wide range of diseases, clinical trials on this drug have nearly come to a complete halt in the United States. Why? Because it was originally developed as an abortion pill.

Clinical trials on the use of RU-486 began as early as 1983 in the United States. Taken in the first nine weeks of a pregnancy, mifepristone was proven to be a relatively safe and effective form of abortion and, since 1988, has been available in Europe as an alternative to vacuum aspiration abortion.

In 1989, Feminist Majority Foundation leaders traveled to France to assess the potential of RU-486. They discovered that this drug had a wide range of potential benefits and, upon their return to the United States, decided to launch a national public education drive. A broad range of research was initiated in areas such as breast cancer, ovarian cancer, brain tumors, Cushing's syndrome, the HIV virus, uterine fibroids, and endometriosis—research that, today, is at a relative standstill.

From the very beginning, antiabortionists have been actively involved in preventing the approval and distribution of RU-486 in the United States. Over and over again they have stepped in and actively involved Congress and the FDA in attempting to put a complete halt to all clinical trials that involve mifepristone, including those that already were showing incredible promise for the treatment of uterine fibroids and endometriosis.

Politics involving this drug have been so hotly debated that seventeen years came and went with little progress toward getting it actually approved by the FDA and available for distribution and further research. Although the American Association for Advancement of Science (AAAS) endorsed the testing of RU-486 in 1991, the debate raged. Although nearly every major scientific and medical organization in this country endorsed the testing of RU-486, the blocking tactics continued.

During all this time, the patent changed hands and now belongs to the Population Council (an international organization concerned with world-wide reproductive health and population growth), several potential manufacturers of the drug have bowed out, and its name eventually reverted back to its scientific name: mifepristone. In 1994 clinical trials began on mifepristone.

By 1995, Dr. Faina Rose announced study results showing that mifepristone inhibits the growth of cancer cells. Dr. David Weiner showed that mifepristone might prevent cell infection and subsequent replication of the HIV virus. By 1996, the Population Council submitted a New Drug Application to the FDA with the FDA Advisory Committee subsequently recommending mifepristone for approval. Four years later, in the fall of 2000, this drug was finally formally approved and released for distribution. Even so, abortion politics and blocking tactics continue as legislators introduce bill after bill into Congress that would block or limit distribution.

While mifepristone has clearly proven to be a safe and effective means of terminating pregnancy during the first nine weeks, this book isn't about abortion. This book is about uterine fibroids. From my perspective, critical research on the viability of mifepristone as an anti-uterine fibroid drug is clearly being blocked by politics that have nothing to do with the science of uterine fibroids; or endometriosis; or breast cancer; or ovarian cancer; or brain tumors; or the HIV virus; or Cushing's syndrome. After reviewing the research and current clinical trial protocols for brain tumors and uterine fibroids, it saddens me a great deal that advances have been so slow and political maneuvers have been so effective in limiting the availability of this drug for research. Early studies are astounding. Brain tumor research alone contains compelling evidence that this drug deserves closer attention.

As for uterine fibroids, a study conducted in 1993 at the University of California, San Diego School of Medicine, watched the progress of ten patients over a period of three months who were given mifepristone daily. At the end of twelve weeks, the mean volume of the women's fibroid uteri decreased by 49 percent. In addition to blocking progesterone action (which is what makes this drug work well for early abortions), mifepristone also blocks estrogen. It is speculated by researchers that mifepristone's combined interference with both progesterone and estrogen is what causes the fibroids to shrink.

Current studies under way are limited in size but do show tremendous promise. Uterine fibroids research currently in progress at the University of Rochester Medical Center has researchers studying the following items:

➤ the rate and degree of regression of fibroids in women taking mifepristone and whether regrowth occurs after stopping the medication
➤ whether symptoms from fibroids are improved in women taking
  mifepristone
➤ whether symptoms from fibroids return after stopping the medication
➤ whether mifepristone is safe when taken at the proposed daily dosage
➤ identifying potential side effects
➤ whether women in the study postpone or avoid surgical treatment for
  their fibroids.

Why should this drug be different from any other used in clinical trials to assess effectiveness in battling disease? Eleanor Smeal, president of
the Feminist Majority, said it best when she stated the following: *"We
should be having a war on cancer . . . not on its [mifepristone's] use for abortion."*
It's truly unfortunate that the mifepristone research addressing a broad
range of diseases has been so limited in the United States. While waiting
for the people in this country (who have the power to make a difference)
to think more intelligently about the far-reaching potential benefits of
mifepristone, there are several dozen people with Cushing's syndrome,
brain tumors, and breast cancer who have been using this drug under
compassionate use protocols. Meanwhile, mifepristone and fibroid tumor
along with endometriosis research in the United States has been slow going. Hopefully, the recent approval of this drug will open doors for additional researchers to take a closer look at this drug for use in future
clinical trials.

Mifepristone Compassionate Use

The Feminist Majority Foundation currently has sole responsibility in the
United States for distributing mifepristone for "compassionate use." While
this drug is now available as an abortificant, the dosage is significantly different from the daily dose taken by patients in the current compassionate
use protocols for their disease. Patients who suffer from serious or life-
threatening diseases and conditions for which no other treatment is available, such as brain tumors, may be eligible for the correct prescriptive
dosage and use of mifepristone under the compassionate use program.

(Last year, I learned that my own sister, who has had two brain tumors removed in her lifetime, might be eligible as a compassionate use patient to receive mifepristone.) For more information on this drug and to learn more about the compassionate use protocol for mifepristone, contact:

Feminist Majority Foundation
1600 Wilson Boulevard, Suite 801
Arlington, VA 22209
(703) 522-2214
http://www.feminist.org

Female Reconstructive Surgery (FRS)

Once upon a time, many years ago and before a doctor by the name of Vicki Hufnagel had her license revoked in California, there was a woman living in Colorado (me) who was desperately seeking information on alternatives to hysterectomy. In my quest for information, one of the many books I purchased was *No More Hysterectomies,* written by Dr. Vicki Hufnagel (c1989) who was practicing medicine, at the time, in Beverly Hills. There were no other books that detailed or offered an alternative surgical solution to the hysterectomy treatment option at that time.

I was amazed. The book seemed like a godsend. This woman was incredible. She could "do it all" and then some and, what's more, she helped author the informed consent laws on hysterectomy for the state of California. This woman was truly remarkable. Could I really bypass a hysterectomy this easily? Why weren't more doctors offering this as an alternative solution? Perhaps it requires special surgical skill? I didn't know the answers to those questions, but I was determined to find out. I called Dr. Hufnagel's office and spoke, at length, to a staff person. She, rather easily, convinced me that female reconstructive surgery (FRS) with Dr. Hufnagel would be the best decision I ever made. So, I scheduled an appointment—for *surgery.*

The plan was simple. I was to fly to California and, in her office, review information and videos on the procedure. Then, I would sign all the necessary paperwork, pay the bill, and undergo surgery. I would return home a "new woman" within a matter of days. There wasn't even a preliminary checkup required, as that would all be taken care of upon my arrival. It sounded too good to be true. I was ecstatic.

At this juncture, I told my husband all about my plans as I knew we would need to make arrangements for additional care of our three children during my absence. He was quite taken aback. Speechless is probably the best way to describe his reaction. Then he read her book. Then he started asking questions. Questions like, "Why is she the only doctor in the world to offer this?" Something didn't seem quite right to him, and I must admit that I had many of the same questions but was simply so thrilled to find an alternative solution to hysterectomy that I deliberately shoved all those questions out of my mind. At his questioning, however, I decided to at least log on to the Internet and check her medical record.

What I found was curious. The Medical Board of California had identified her physician/license status as "decision stayed." What did this mean? I didn't know. But, I wanted to find out. I called the Medical Board of California and was told that they could not disclose any information over the telephone. "*But I have surgery scheduled!*" I whined. "*Is there anything at **all** you can tell me?*"

The person on the other end of the line hesitated. "*I'm not supposed to do this. You didn't hear it from me. Her license is being revoked. Run, don't walk. That's all I will say.*"

I was stunned. I didn't know what any of it meant. What should I do? At that time she still had her license. If whatever she was doing were so bad surely they would have at least suspended it or something, wouldn't they? Surely they wouldn't allow her to continue performing surgery on unsuspecting women if they were revoking her license? (*I've since learned that the answer to this question is, yes, they would. It's called "due process"— while the case is under review or moving through the court system, the physician may have the right to continue practicing medicine.*)

After much discussion with my husband, I decided to call Dr. Hufnagel's office and ask to speak directly with her. I would reassure her that my surgery was still scheduled and that I had every intention of keeping that appointment, but that I simply needed to hear from her what, exactly, was going on in California with her license. It sounded like a good plan.

So, I dialed the number. At first, the staff person on the other end of the telephone insisted that Dr. Hufnagel was too busy to speak with me.

Huh? Too busy? "*But I'm scheduled for surgery with her. What do you mean she's too busy to speak to me? I've never even met this woman and yet I've, on faith, scheduled surgery with her but she's too busy to speak to me?*"

The answer was yes. She insisted that Dr. Hufnagel was simply too busy and that all my questions would be answered once I arrived in California for my appointment.

"In that case, I will have to cancel the appointment. I am not flying all the way to California for surgery with a doctor who won't even answer my questions or speak to me beforehand."

She put me on hold. The next person that picked up the line was Dr. Hufnagel. *"I understand you have some questions?"*

I thanked her for taking the time to speak with me, as my comfort zone needed reassurance from the physician who would be doing the surgery. She told me that all my questions would be answered when I arrived and that I would be a "new woman." Then, I asked her my question.

"Dr. Hufnagel, I do have surgery scheduled and do intend to keep that appointment, but I was checking on your license with the medical board and was told that your license is being revoked. Can you tell me what that is all about?"

What happened next was completely unanticipated by me. She began ranting and raving with such venom that it was all I could do to continue holding the phone to listen to it all. This was the doctor that I was actually going to let cut me open. Without ever meeting her first. What in the world was I thinking? Just how desperate had I become?

I didn't learn until later what was going on with Dr. Hufnagel and the medical board in California, but my experience strongly suggested it was not enhancing her ability to communicate professionally with her patients. How was it enhancing/hindering her ability to perform surgery competently? I didn't know and I didn't want to find out.

It has been many years since this incident, and it has taken me some time to unravel it all. But, ultimately, this experience taught me more lessons about medicine and doctors than you could ever imagine. It gave new meaning to the phrase *If it seems to be too good to be true, then it probably is.*

So what is FRS anyway? I think of Female Reconstructive Surgery like this: Any and every body part involved in your reproductive system requiring medical attention will be fixed without performing a hysterectomy. Removing fibroids, endometriosis, and/or adenomyosis, performing bladder resuspension, draining cysts, repairing fallopian tubes, and reshaping your labia are typical of FRS.

This is what I later discovered about Vicki Hufnagel's run-in with the California Medical Board. After complaints were filed against Dr. Hufnagel, the California Medical Board conducted an investigation and in 1987 brought disciplinary charges against her including allegations of gross negligence and incompetence in treatment of more than ten patients and false and fraudulent billing. Throughout 1987 and 1988, hearings were held before an administrative law judge (ALJ) and legal briefs were submitted and oral arguments heard. A proposed decision by the ALJ was not adopted by the medical board, which independently decided the case with more stringent consequences for Hufnagel. In 1989 the medical board found sufficient grounds to order revocation of Hufnagel's medical license in six of the patient cases, suspension in four of the cases, and probation in two of the cases. While Hufnagel continues to argue otherwise, the board specifically stated in its decision that her belief that too many unnecessary hysterectomies are performed had no bearing on its decision.

The disciplinary action ordered by the board was not actually carried out at that time because Hufnagel petitioned the California courts to review the case and the courts granted a stay of the board's orders pending court review. Therefore, during this period Hufnagel was still practicing medicine, and I would have gone under her knife for female reconstructive surgery had it not been for my husband's healthy skepticism and my checking her credentials. It was not until 1996 that the California court finally found the penalty of revocation appropriate under "the totality of the circumstances." No further stay was granted and after nine years of legal proceedings Hufnagel finally had to surrender her license. Her further attempts to get the California Supreme Court and the U.S. Supreme Court to review her case were rejected. You can read on Hufnagel's website www.drhufnagel.com her account of these events and her theories about what motivated them. She also asserts that she may reapply for her California medical license in 1999; however, as of this writing the medical board's public records indicate that the revocation is still in effect. Copies of the proceedings can be purchased from the California medical board for a copying fee.

California reports all actions taken against physicians to the National Practitioner Database, which in turn sends out notifications to all states where the physician is licensed to practice medicine. In addition, the Medical Board of California reports all final actions taken against physicians to the Federation of State Medical Boards. With both of these actions, all states are notified whenever there is negative activity on a physician's license in the state of California.

During the time Hufnagel's case was in progress, she had licenses to practice medicine in Hawaii and New York. New York has since revoked her license. As of this writing, she is still licensed in Hawaii.

Was Hufnagel Singled Out?

Before believing the cries from Vicki Hufnagel that she was "singled out" by her peers, please be sure to review the latest annual license revocation information found in the Summary of Board Actions found on line at:
   http://www.fsmb.org/
   In 1999, there were 1,664 physician license revocations. 207 were from California.
   Just to ensure that 1996 wasn't an unusual year with only Vicki Hufnagel losing her license, I made a few inquiries. According to the Federation of State Medical Boards, in 1996 there were 1,607 physician license revocations throughout the United States—177 in California alone.

The public records for Ms. Hufnagel's case in the state of California indicate there were real victims. People. Women who trusted her just as I did—and then some. While Ms. Hufnagel states repeatedly that the license revocation was part of a campaign by the male patriarchal medical world to silence her constant attacks regarding unnecessary hysterectomy surgery in the United States, the findings in the official records suggest otherwise.

While I may agree with Ms. Hufnagel's assessment that there is a very real patriarchal medical world that has openly placed a woman's uterus on the auction block of medicine while making only limited attempts at researching alternative solutions (to hysterectomy) that are more reasonable, I do not necessarily agree that she was a victim of "speaking out" against her peers. I've learned, over time, that many, many doctors speak out and seek out alternative solutions for their patients. While finding one of these wonderful doctors may, at times, seem difficult, it is not impossible. (See chapter 8; *Making a Decision*) for more information on how to go about finding a **licensed** physician who has never been disciplined.)

I can never stress enough the importance of doing your homework in researching the background of the physician chosen to perform surgery on your body. In Hufnagel's case, there are many women who will readily communicate to you that she is a fine surgeon and her turn of licensure events is pure peer persecution for her anti-hysterectomy activities. As a result, many women travel to Mexico for surgery (where Ms. Hufnagel continues to provide FRS).

The court records do not support those claims, however, and are an excellent example of how critical it is for each of us to take the necessary steps and precautions to verify the credentials of our physicians.

Seven

Related Health Issues

In choosing a course of treatment for uterine fibroids, you may find the task at hand complicated by any number of related health issues. This chapter takes a look at the interrelated health problems that may or may not be present along with uterine fibroids. Although physicians often look at these items as separate issues and treat them separately from uterine fibroids, they can have an impact on the overall recommendation for treatment received from a physician. Related health issues briefly covered in this chapter include:

➤ adenomyosis
➤ cancer
➤ dysplasia
➤ endometriosis
➤ hyperplasia
➤ ovarian cysts
➤ polyps
➤ sexual dysfunction
➤ uterine prolapse

Adenomyosis

Adenomyosis is a benign disease of the uterus that can and does produce symptoms very similar to uterine fibroids. It is the growth of endometrial tissue from the uterine lining into the myometrium and is sometimes called "internal endometriosis." The endometrial cells penetrate deep into the walls of the uterus, enlarging the uterus as the disease progresses. Due to this uterine enlargement, this disease is often misdiagnosed as uterine fibroids during pelvic examination and is a prime example of why it is so important for women to seek out additional diagnostic measures for a more complete picture of their uterine condition.

Currently, the typical method of diagnosing adenomyosis is through hysterectomy. Other ways in which adenomyosis can be diagnosed are through MRI (magnetic resonance imaging) and transvaginal ultrasound. When fibroids are present, however, both of these methods can prove difficult in distinguishing the fibroids from adenomyosis. In recent years, advances in differentiating adenomyosis on MRI have been made, and this is now considered one of the most accurate ways one can diagnose adenomyosis prior to treatment.

Even with imaging advances, the only known definitive cure for this disease is hysterectomy. Research is moving forward somewhat, however, as a few physicians have attempted to remove parts of the uterus containing adenomyosis disease and then to reconstruct the uterus. In the cases where this has been attempted, patients are reporting that their bleeding is back to normal menstrual cycles and their pain has dissipated. This treatment option has a long road to travel before we know enough about the long-term outcome to say that it is truly an option for women with adenomyosis.

Another area of adenomyosis research involves uterine artery embolization. Because approximately 50 percent of women who have adenomyosis also have uterine fibroids, many of these women found themselves seeking out uterine artery embolization as a treatment option for their fibroids. Results were quite positive as both the adenomyosis and uterine fibroids reduced in bulk with this procedure. Symptoms of pain and bleeding were resolved and, as a result, additional research was launched to determine whether or not uterine artery embolization would be a viable treatment option for women with ONLY adenomyosis. Early results are showing 90 percent improvement in symptoms and, although this treatment option also has a long road to travel, it certainly is looking like a very promising option for women with adenomyosis.

Cancer

Throughout this book, statistical risks of varying types of cancer have been presented and discussed. Occasionally, while seeking out a treatment option for fibroids, diagnostic tests can reveal an entirely different picture for a woman. This issue was brought to my attention during the last two years when, many times over, women seeking out information on uterine artery embolization as a treatment option for their symptomatic uterine fibroids were directed to go back to their physician and ask about an endometrial biopsy. The heavy bleeding these women were experiencing simply required a closer look to ensure that hyperplasia or endometrial cancer wasn't present before they ventured down the road to making a treatment decision.

Several times, women reported back to me that they were shocked to discover they had endometrial cancer. They knew they had fibroids. They knew they were experiencing heavy bleeding over a very long period of time (many months/years). They knew they did not want a hysterectomy and, therefore, chose not to return to their gynecologist for follow-up care after receiving the standard recommendation for hysterectomy. What they didn't know was that heavy prolonged bleeding of this nature could be indicative of other, more serious problems than uterine fibroids. Although these women chose to finally seek out care again so that they could undergo uterine artery embolization, they ultimately ended up with hysterectomy and chemotherapy.

Although uterine fibroids may be present in your body, symptoms that you experience may or may not be the direct result of those uterine fibroids. Appropriate diagnostic tests administered regularly during the "watchful waiting" phase of fibroid growth and development is critical. If your doctor recommends a hysterectomy and you don't believe that to be an appropriate treatment option, do not confuse your disagreement with your physician with the need to be appropriately tested on a regular basis. Annual pap smears are still an absolute must as are endometrial biopsies when heavy bleeding is present.

Once a gynecological cancer is diagnosed, most of the treatment options in this book are a moot point. Even so, you might be surprised to learn that there are many women diagnosed with gynecological cancer who are not interested in hearing about hysterectomy as a treatment option. Reasons for avoiding hysterectomy even when cancer is present range from wanting to have another child to not wanting sexual function altered by surgery, to believing they can naturally treat their disease, to simply not wanting to be cut open. They would rather die first. Of course, most of these women don't actually believe that death will happen to them.

Other reasons might include simply not wanting to trade their current quality of life for an unknown, potentially lesser quality of life after hysterectomy.

Anyone who has watched and experienced the death of a loved one from any of the gynecological cancers will tell you one thing: If cancer is diagnosed, please get the appropriately recommended treatment. Even if it is hysterectomy. Learn as much as you can about your condition and work with your doctors to resolve this illness.

Dysplasia

The Pap smear that you undergo annually was designed to determine the presence of cervical dysplasia and cervical cancer. Cervical dysplasia is simply the abnormal growth of cell tissue on the cervix. It is not cancer. It is, however, a precancerous condition that, if left untreated, can progress to cervical cancer.

Even though fibroids may be present, it is still critical for you to undergo an annual Pap smear. It doesn't matter how large or small your fibroids are or where they are located in/on your uterus; all women (even those who've undergone hysterectomy that resulted in the removal of their cervix—although the cervix may no longer be present, abnormal cells can still develop in the vagina) should have an annual Pap smear. Although at least one physician told me that the presence of large fibroids would skew the test results from a Pap smear, his commentary couldn't have been further from the truth. The presence of fibroids is not an indication that you should forgo the annual Pap smear.

Treatment options for dysplasia include cryotherapy, LEEP (loop electrosurgical excision procedure), laser therapy, and cone biopsy. Cryotherapy freezes and kills the abnormal cervical cells; LEEP involves a hot electrical current that, with the use of a wire loop, slices away the abnormal cells; laser therapy burns away abnormal cells; and cone biopsy involves the surgical removal of a portion of the outside of the cervix and the inside canal of the cervix. Cure rates for all of these treatments run at about 95 percent.

While hysterectomy is sometimes recommended to patients with advanced dysplasia, it is generally not necessary except as a last resort when treatment has failed repeatedly and/or the condition progresses to cervical cancer.

Endometriosis

Endometriosis is the growth of tissue from the endometrium into parts of the pelvis where it does not belong. When it grows, this tissue can be found throughout the abdominal cavity and typically engulfs the internal organs. The result of all this unwanted and misdirected tissue growth can be extremely painful periods, chronic pelvic pain, pain with sex, painful bowel movements, and constant backache (to name just a few symptoms!). Those symptoms combined with uterine fibroids make for a very low quality of life for the woman who is unfortunate enough to experience both at the same time.

Endometriosis and resulting symptoms are heavily impacted by a woman's menstrual cycle. The ebb and flow of the hormonal tide in a month does seem to play a role in both growth of endometriosis and the severity of symptoms experienced.

There is no "cure" for endometriosis, and even hysterectomy cannot prevent the return of this disease within the pelvis. Treatment options are limited and generally involve progesterone, Gonadotropin-releasing hormone (GnRH) agonists, or birth-control pills. Several extremely experienced laparoscopic surgeons have reported excellent results with laparoscopic removal of endometriosis tissue—but these skilled surgeons are a rarity.

When fibroids are present along with endometriosis, this presents a treatment dilemma. Use of hormonal remedies is problematic as these very remedies that might help with endometriosis may also cause the fibroids to grow, except for GnRH, which, of course, cannot be used for more than six months. With uterine artery embolization research, there was tremendous hope that this procedure might be beneficial to patients with endometriosis. Alas, it is not. In fact, UAE is not recommended as a treatment option for women with endometriosis because it simply does not resolve the pain issues and may, quite possibly, contribute to infections requiring hysterectomy.

While there has been some endometriosis research, truly it is limited. Early studies looking at mifepristone as an option were extremely promising but were discontinued when researchers found it impossible to obtain the drug.

Clearly, we need more research. In writing this book, I was overwhelmed by the sheer quantity of hysterectomy research and seriously underwhelmed by the lack of research that looked at cause and effect. In all areas of female reproductive health there is a serious deficiency in scientific research that would give us any answers as to the "why" of these diseases. Without the "why," we can only continue to rely on surgery and limited treatment methods in an effort to fend off disease progression. This is far from optimal.

For a more comprehensive and thoroughly researched discussion of endometriosis, I highly recommend the *Women's Encyclopedia of Natural Medicine,* by Dr. Tori Hudson. Treatment options are truly limited with endometriosis, but a naturopathic approach has proven successful for many women. Dr. Hudson's book presents a balanced discussion of both naturopathic and conventional medical approaches that may prove helpful to women with endometriosis.

Hyperplasia

Hyperplasia is the excessive growth of abnormal cells in the endometrial lining. High levels of estrogen and a complete absence of progesterone causes these cells to grow and, over time, the lining can become quite thick. At some point, the cells become quite fragile and constant and/or unpredictable bleeding is the result. Hyperplasia is a noncancerous condition that is easily diagnosed with a D&C or endometrial biopsy.

Hyperplasia is generally stated to be "with atypia" (atypical hyperplasia) or "without atypia" (simple hyperplasia), and this distinction can make a world of difference in terms of treatment options. Just as dysplasia has the potential to develop into cervical cancer, atypical hyperplasia has the potential to develop into endometrial (uterine) cancer.

Hyperplasia is the result of hormonal imbalances (just like fibroids!), and women who are diagnosed with hyperplasia all lack appropriate progesterone levels. The first line of defense for hyperplasia is progesterone pills, as this is an easy way to increase a woman's progesterone levels and prevent the hyperplasia from progressing. If this treatment along with a D&C doesn't work to stop hyperplasia from developing into endometrial cancer, it would then be appropriate to turn to hysterectomy.

It shouldn't be a surprise to you that many women with uterine fibroids at some point end up with hyperplasia if their fibroids and resulting symptoms are left untreated. Hormonal imbalances that incite fibroid growth seem to incite fast multiplication of cell growth of the endometrial lining as well. If hyperplasia and uterine fibroids are both part of your diagnosis and abnormal bleeding is a major symptom, treating the hyperplasia first with progesterone may well bring the bleeding under control, thus, allowing you to postpone treatment for your uterine fibroids until they become symptomatic enough on their own to warrant action.

Ovarian Cysts

Ovarian cysts and your treatment options can be almost as difficult to understand and frustrating as uterine fibroids. Ovarian cysts develop from the collection of fluid within the ovary—which is normally a solid organ. Cysts are extremely common among women. The vast majority of ovarian cysts are benign and go away all by themselves. Some cysts are persistent, however, and others can be cancerous. Transvaginal ultrasound can give your physician a fairly accurate diagnosis of which type of cyst has developed, lending a much better idea of the appropriate treatment option.

Certainly, combined with uterine fibroids, these two diseases can present a bit of a dilemma for the patient and physician alike in terms of what course of action might be best for the individual. Too often I receive email from women with benign ovarian cysts who, because they also happen to have fibroids, are told they need a hysterectomy—even when the fibroids are not causing them any problems whatsoever and the cysts could be treated with less invasive and less drastic measures. Undergoing a hysterectomy simply because one has cysts certainly increases your surgical risks, perhaps unnecessarily. If your gynecologist recommends a hysterectomy to go along with treating your ovarian cyst, it might be wise to *get a second opinion!*

If ovarian cysts are a part of your medical condition, reading *A Gynecologist's Second Opinion,* by Dr. William Parker, may provide you with a strong understanding of this common gynecological problem and offer insight into the measures you can take to treat this condition and retain your organs.

Polyps

Polyps are teardrop-shaped folds of the endometrial lining that develop and hang from the endometrium. These growths develop when there is an absence of progesterone and an ever-increasing amount of estrogen. Typically, polyps keep good company with hyperplasia. Again, abnormal bleeding can be a sign that polyps have developed, but the good news is that they are usually quite easily removed in your doctor's office with the assistance of a hysteroscope.

Depending on the growth and development of the endometrium and the polyp(s), a D&C could also be performed or, in some cases, resectioning of the polyp may be needed while you are under anesthesia in an outpatient hospital facility. As with hyperplasia, polyps are quite common growths in women with uterine fibroids. If abnormal bleeding is present, treatment of the polyps may resolve the problem. Even so, hormonal imbalances clearly exist and may well cause the development of more polyps at a later time if hormonal treatment is not sought in an attempt to balance the lack of progesterone.

Prolapse

Weaknesses in the vagina and the support ligaments holding the bladder, rectum, and uterus in place can cause the descent, or dropping, of an organ into the vagina. This condition is called prolapse and can be quite an uncomfortable situation. The constant feeling that something is falling down and out the vagina (indeed it is!) can be quite painful and result in low back pain as well as painful sexual intercourse.

Prolapse is a common aftereffect of hysterectomy, typically occurring five to ten years after the procedure, but is mainly considered to be one result of childbirth. During childbirth, as with hysterectomy, the pelvic structural ligaments are sometimes damaged creating a weakness in pelvic structural support. This in turn, and over time, leads to prolapse.

There are two types of prolapse: uterine prolapse and vaginal prolapse. Uterine prolapse refers to the uterus dropping down into the vagina. It typically drops in stages until, at some point in time, it actually appears at the entrance to the vagina. Vaginal prolapse refers to the dropping of other organs into the vagina, and each one of these organs has its own name for this occurrence.

Type of Vaginal Prolapse	Description
Cystocele	Part of the bladder drops into the vagina.
Cystourethrocele	Combination of bladder and urethra drops into the vagina.
Enterocele	A loop of intestine drops between the rectum and the vagina.
Rectocele	Wall of the rectum protrudes into the vagina.
Urethrocele	The urethra drops into the vagina.

Resulting symptoms from vaginal prolapse include bladder weakness with urine leakage, urinary tract infections, a feeling of downward pressure in the vagina, pressure on the rectum, and inability to completely empty all fecal matter.

Dealing with prolapse can range from using a pessary (a rubber device inserted into the vagina to support the uterus in place), to surgery that repairs the muscles and ligaments and repositions the pelvic organs, to vaginal hysterectomy. The presence of fibroids can certainly complicate matters and place even more undue pressure on the downward advance of a woman's organs. On the other hand, fibroids that are quite large can serve, in some ways, as a blocking mechanism to prolapse. Either way, the situation is most likely to be extremely uncomfortable.

Surgery to repair any prolapse may require surgery to remove uterine fibroids at the same time. Under these circumstances, a urogynecologist—a gynecologist with advanced training in urology, specifically treatment of incontinence and prolapse—may be the best type of physician to consult. The following organization is available as a resource to help you locate a urogynecologist:

American Urogynecologic Society
2025 M Street NW, Suite 800
Washington, DC 20036
(202) 367-1167
http://www.augs.org

Sexual Dysfunction

According to a study published in 1999 on Sexual Dysfunction in the United States (JAMA 1999;281:537-544), as many as 43 percent of all women in the United States experience some form of sexual dysfunction. Before we can even begin to look at the issue of sexual dysfunction potentially occurring as the direct result of a pelvic surgical procedure, however, we must first recognize that there is quite clearly a problem in this nation with female sexual function that desperately demands attention. The information gathered for this particular study used a national probability sample of 1,749 women and 1,410 men aged eighteen to fifty-nine years.

Although the results written about in this study didn't identify prior surgical procedures that any of the women may have possibly undergone, it was still an astounding collection of data filled with valuable nuggets of information. Some key points:

➤ As a woman ages, sexual problems tend to *decrease*—with the exception of those who report trouble with lubrication.

➤ Married women (and men) are associated with a *decreased* risk of experiencing sexual problems.

➤ Nonmarried women are one and a half times *more likely* to have climax problems and sexual anxiety.

➤ Women with college degrees report higher sexual desire, fewer problems achieving orgasm, less sexual pain, and less sexual anxiety than women who have not graduated from high school.

➤ Overall, women AND men with lower education levels report *less* pleasurable sexual experience and *raised* levels of sexual anxiety.

➤ Black women tend to have *higher* rates of low sexual desire and experience *less* pleasure compared to white women.

➤ White women are *more likely* to experience sexual pain than black women.

➤ Those who experience emotional or stress-related problems are *more likely* to experience sexual dysfunction.

➤ Lower household income puts women at *higher* risk for sexual dysfunction.

➤ Women with low sexual activity (fewer than five lifetime partners and limited masturbation) are at *higher* risk for low sexual desire and arousal disorders.

➤ Women reporting same-sex activity are *not at higher risk* than women with male partners.

➤ Arousal disorder appears to be *highly* associated in women who were sexual victims through adult-child contact or forced sexual contact.

➤ Sexual dysfunction is most common among *young* women.

As I read this study, the sheer numbers of women in this country not enjoying a healthy sex life free of sexual dysfunction nearly blew my socks off. But wait, this isn't the only study that's been done; others have estimated that up to 76 percent of women have complaints of sexual dysfunction which include: decreased libido, vaginal dryness, pain with intercourse, decreased genital sensation, and difficulty/inability to achieve orgasm. Perhaps *half* of all women over the age of forty have sexual complaints. Yikes! That's a lot of women.

In reviewing the sexual dysfunction studies that have been done on women who've undergone hysterectomy, something startling pops to the surface. Study after study show sexual dysfunction for women both pre- and post-hysterectomy at lower levels than the national population samples. Due to the impact of disease that often brings on depression, abnormal bleeding, pain, and sexual discomfort, one would think that the number of women reporting some element of sexual dysfunction prior to hysterectomy would be HIGHER than the general population studies. Instead, hysterectomy studies all show levels of dysfunction for these women both before and after their hysterectomy as being LOWER than the general population. Clearly, something is wrong with either the general population studies or the hysterectomy and sexual functioning research. As I looked over the data collection methodologies for both types of studies, I determined that time and again the collection methods and questions asked of women in the hysterectomy studies were limited in scope and did not recognize or inquire about the full range of sexual dysfunction that potentially exists in the female population. If only four questions regarding sexual function are asked of women undergoing hysterectomy, are their answers really going to provide a comprehensive picture of these women both before and after hysterectomy? Without a baseline reading of what sexual function was like for these women prior to the onset of disease, are pre- and post-hysterectomy data comparison and analysis truly relevant?

The flaws that exist in the hysterectomy and sexual function studies are abundant. Data analysis is typically incomplete and inconclusive and, as a result, I have a terrible time trying to understand the doctors who tell patients, "Research shows that a hysterectomy has a positive impact on sexual function." This answer is frequently served up as a reassuring and definitive response to the question "How will my sex life be impacted by a hysterectomy—will it cause sexual dysfunction?" From my viewpoint, the research that would truly answer that question has simply not even been approached yet.

To develop a better understanding of what, exactly, may be wrong with these studies, and to acquire a broader understanding of female sexual function, the information in this section is broken down into the following four subsections:

➤ psychological and physiological characteristics of female sexual function
➤ female sexual dysfunction classifications

➤ potential impact of pelvic surgery
➤ sexual healing

Female Sexual Function

A woman's sexual response cycle is made up of four stages:

➤ excitement
➤ plateau
➤ orgasm
➤ resolution

During the first stage, *excitement,* blood flow to the pelvic region increases (blood vessels in the vagina, labia, and clitoris all dilate, causing blood to rush into the area) and the uterus becomes elevated. The vagina expands by about three inches in diameter and one inch in length. With the second stage, *plateau,* the uterus elevates and enlarges even more—typically expanding to nearly twice its normal size. During the third stage, *orgasm,* the uterus contracts as do the muscles surrounding the vagina and rectum. The very strength of these contractions during the third stage may contribute to the overall intensity of orgasm that many women experience. The fourth stage, *resolution,* is the ramp down to the presexual arousal stage. However, some women who are able to sustain sexual excitement during the resolution stage actually report additional orgasms.

While the clitoris is a major source of stimulation and sexual pleasure that contributes to the four stages of female sexual function, the uterus and the blood flow generated to the entire pelvic region are also factors that contribute to a woman's overall sexual pleasure during sex. Even so, not all women are cognizant of uterine or vaginal contractions and do not sense the changes that occur in these regions during sexual intercourse. For these women, orgasms are said to be primarily clitoral.

Why do some women experience only clitoral orgasms while others can sense vaginal or uterine-contraction orgasms? Is one type of orgasm better than the other? Considering the lack of research into the physiological aspects of female sexual function, these are impossible questions to answer with any true knowledge or accuracy of detail. Regardless, the level of interest you have in sex as well as the type of orgasms YOU experience (and consider an enjoyable aspect of your Quality of Life that you don't want altered!) can play a major role in the decision-making process for selecting a treatment option for uterine fibroids.

Female Sexual Dysfunction Classifications

Masters and Johnson were the first to lay out the basic foundation in 1966 for what we know about female sexual response, but very few studies focusing on female anatomy and physiology in relation to sexual disorders have been done since that time. In fact, only within the last couple of years have researchers stepped up to the plate in larger numbers and started to look at this issue.

Ways to diagnose sexual dysfunction have evolved over time, and there are currently six classifications that the American Psychiatric Association uses today to identify female sexual dysfunction:

1. hypoactive sexual desire disorder
2. sexual aversion disorder
3. female sexual arousal disorders
4. female orgasmic disorders
5. dyspareunia (painful sexual intercourse)
6. vaginismus

The biggest problem with this particular set of diagnosis classifications is that sexual therapists and psychiatrists have pretty much always been the therapeutic group doing the diagnosis and developing the definitions. There seems to be a distinct lack of clinical, physical markers that differentiate each of the categories. Confusion over the definitions and what, precisely, is included in each category is apparent by the variety of interpretations that abound in the medical literature.

In 1998, this classification system was redesigned by a multidisciplinary panel of experts (urology, gynecology, nursing, pharmacology, psychiatry, psychology, and rehabilitative medicine). It was important to this team of experts to redefine and classify female sexual disorders in a way that would create uniformity of terms and standards and still allow room for potential growth in laboratory and clinical research.

The classifications for female sexual dysfunction overlap and are often accompanied by the additional problem of depression. While both phys-

Female Sexual Dysfunction Classifications and Definitions

1. **Hypoactive sexual desire disorder.** Persistent or recurring deficiency (or absence) of sexual fantasies/thoughts and/or desire for or receptivity to sexual activity, which causes personal distress.
   a. **Sexual aversion disorder.** Persistent or recurring phobic aversion to, and avoidance of, sexual contact with a sexual partner, which causes personal distress.
2. **Sexual arousal disorder.** Persistent or recurring inability to attain or to maintain sufficient sexual excitement, thereby causing personal distress. It may be experienced as a lack of subjective excitement or a lack of genital (lubrication/swelling) or other somatic responses.
3. **Orgasmic disorder.** Persistent or recurrent difficulty, delay in, or absence of attaining orgasm following sufficient sexual stimulation and arousal, causing personal distress.
4. **Sexual pain disorders**
   a. **Dyspareunia.** Recurrent or persistent genital pain associated with sexual intercourse.
   b. **Vaginismus.** Recurrent or persistent involuntary spasm of the musculature of the outer third of the vagina that interferes with vaginal penetration, causing personal distress.
   c. **Other sexual pain disorders.** Recurrent or persistent genital pain induced by noncoital sexual stimulation.

iological and psychological factors may play a role in sexual dysfunction, there is an ongoing debate among researchers as to which issue contributes the most to a patient's condition. Laura Berman, a psychotherapist from the Boston Women's Sexual Health Clinic, states that only 20 percent of her patients have purely psychological problems that drive their sexual dysfunction. The remaining 80 percent have either a combination of physiological and psychological problems or purely physiological problems.

Research on sexual dysfunction is evolving with each new study that's completed, and it is hoped that this new classification system will be better able to evolve along with the ever-emerging information that is building in our body of knowledge.

Potential Impact of Pelvic Surgery

The physiological aspects of a woman's sexual function are currently very poorly understood. Although a great deal of research is under way, the clinical methods for measuring female sexual function are still in laboratory design stages. Until more is known about the blood flow to each organ and area of the pelvic region, muscular contractions, and how it all works together with the central nervous system to send signals of pleasure to the brain during sex, we can't know for certain how any one surgical procedure of the pelvic region may impact/influence sexual dysfunction in any given woman.

It certainly seems reasonable to expect that removing the uterus would have a serious impact on women who are sensitive to uterine contractions but, perhaps, would be less of an issue for women who are not. Removing the cervix and thereby possibly shortening the vagina could, very well, create vaginal pain where none existed previously. What about the broad range of interwoven nerves and blood vessels that fill the pelvic region that are connected with the brain as thoughts of desire and arousal stimulate the flow of blood and sensitivity to the region? What if those nerves or blood vessels are damaged in some way during a procedure, thereby making it impossible for the pelvic region to even receive sexual signals from the brain and vice versa?

For far too long, hysterectomy and sexual function studies have focused on the psychological aspects of treatment outcome. Although this focus has its own level of validity based on the very high numbers of women who experience depression after a hysterectomy (43 to 80 percent: Bernstein 1997), it doesn't address the very real aspect of a surgical procedure altering the basic physiology of a woman's reproductive system.

"I never dreamed a hysterectomy would affect my entire being so much. Before my surgery, my spouse and I were having great sex; now it seems as though I couldn't care less if we ever had sex. I do feel like I want to be close to him, but orgasm is a rarity for me now. My doctor made me feel like it was all in my head, but I don't really think so. I feel such an overwhelming sadness now; I just want my life back, my sex life, my body, even my PMS! I feel like it's too late, it's all been taken out and there is nothing I can do about it."—Dolly

The following are some of the risks uniquely associated with various procedures that are used in the treatment of uterine fibroids. This is by no means a complete list, and one should always consider the possibility that ANY type of pelvic surgery has the potential to impact sexual function.

Total Hysterectomy   With a total hysterectomy, the uterus is removed and the cervix and upper portion of the vagina are severed. This generally creates a shortening of the vagina, diminished elasticity, and reduced lubrication—all of which can make sexual intercourse extremely painful. Improper closure of the vaginal cuff can lead to even more painful conditions.

When the cervix is removed, a large portion of the uterovaginal plexus (an interwoven network of blood vessels and nerves) goes with it. Most of the nerve supply to the uterus is concentrated around the cervix. (Indeed, some women need cervical stimulation for orgasm.) Removal of the cervix and uterus could very well negatively impact the sensory information the brain receives.

During a total hysterectomy, in order to dissect and remove the uterus and cervix, clamps are used very close to the ureters. This may contribute to bladder dysfunction, which can cause additional distress during sex.

Subtotal Hysterectomy   Retention of the cervix decreases the level of surgical impact on the vagina and uterovaginal plexus, and ureter complications are much less frequent with the supracervical hysterectomy. When the cervix is retained, the ligaments that support the pelvic floor are not cut but remain intact. The vagina is not shortened, and vaginal lubrication problems are reported less often. Although removal of the uterus may create a decrease in blood flow and a definite loss of pleasurable feelings related to uterine contractions experienced by some women, internal orgasms related to cervical stimulation remain.

Hysterectomy with Bilateral Salpingo-Oophorectomy (BSO)   In addition to the items listed above for hysterectomy, removing the ovaries presents its own set of problems. The ovaries produce estrogen and testosterone and whenever there is deficiency in those hormones, a woman's sexual dysfunction is bound to increase. Estrogen contributes to vaginal lubrication and without it, women experience dry, painful intercourse. Testosterone plays a huge role in desire and arousal and without it, well, women just aren't much interested in sex. While hormone replacement therapy is available for estrogen and testosterone, finding the right dosage as well as avoiding side effects is a very real struggle for a great many women after hysterectomy with BSO.

Uterine Artery Embolization   Because all elements of the reproductive system and all genitalia are kept intact with uterine artery embolization, early considerations of sexual dysfunction as a result of this procedure were nonexistent. However, a recent case was published that discussed the impact of embolizing the cervical branch of the uterine artery—something that is commonly done during UAE. Loss of blood flow to the cervical branch of the uterine artery may have an impact on the uterovaginal plexus and, therefore, may injure the very nerves that allow a woman to experience uterine contractions and internal orgasm. Selectively bypassing the cervical branch of the uterine artery is not always possible and can be extremely difficult to determine. Until further studies are done and more women share their experiences of sexual function/dysfunction post-UAE with their physicians, we can only speculate on the potential for this complication to occur.

Sexual Healing

In addition to pelvic surgery, a variety of other factors can contribute to inadequate blood flow to the pelvic region. Poor circulation, heart disease, diabetes, high cholesterol, smoking, diet, lack of exercise, and a variety of drugs (Zoloft, Prozac, Sertraline, Serafem, etc.) can all contribute to sexual dysfunction. Inadequate blood flow as a result of any of these items can contribute to lack of orgasm, decreased orgasm, and vaginal dryness.

Improving your dietary habits, exercising or increasing your exercise levels, and developing better health habits can be a first line of defense when it comes to increasing blood flow to the pelvic region and enhancing sexual satisfaction. You may not be able to change what occurs as a result of a medical procedure, but you can help your body out by taking these healthy measures to improve your blood flow—as well as your state of mind. After all, exercising produces endorphins that make us "feel good" and, as a result, help us to cope better with the physical limitations at hand.

Vaginal dryness and/or lack of desire are issues directly related to insufficient hormonal levels of estrogen and testosterone. If these problems

UAE and Sexual Dysfunction: A Very Personal Story

As a result of my own UAE, I experienced orgasmic disorder related to the loss of internal orgasms. I subsequently posted that information and my experiences with it in **My Journal** on the http://www.uterinefibroids.com website. As a result, about a dozen women wrote to me sharing their own stories of sexual dysfunction after UAE. It was this information, shared with researchers, that led to the analysis of blood flow and embolization technique that may/may not have contributed to this condition. By speaking up and talking to my physicians about sex and my concerns about altered blood flow with UAE both before and after uterine artery embolization, analysis and review occurred very quickly, potentially saving many women from experiencing similar sexual dysfunction as a result.

Unfortunately, 75 percent of all women express some level of fear in broaching the topic of sex with their physicians. Consequently, physicians who treat us learn very little about female sexual function in their practice and know even less about how to treat us for sexual dysfunction. Two things need to change: 1) women need to overcome their fear and embarrassment and open their mouths and share, share, share, and 2) physicians need to create an environment of open communication that is nonjudgmental and allows for discussion of this topic during a clinical visit.

plague you, ask your doctor to do hormonal testing that includes a blood test of serum-free testosterone and serum DHEA. If these are low, or even on the lower range of the normal scale, prescribing these hormones might be helpful.

Struggling with the outcome of sexual dysfunction after a medical procedure can be traumatic. An open and supportive spouse/sexual partner can be a wonderful individual in whom to confide. In many ways, working with this individual can be instrumental in helping you to overcome whatever areas of dysfunction you experience and can, ultimately, lead to a stronger personal bond with someone you love very much. It can also result in some interesting experimentation with sex that, perhaps, you've never considered before and also, perhaps, help to enhance your sexual function.

Seeking out professional counseling for support and guidance can also contribute to sexual healing. The American Association of Sex Educators,

Counselors and Therapists (AASECT) can help you locate a certified sexuality counselor or therapist who practices in your region. To receive a list of certified practitioners through the postal service, send a stamped, self-addressed envelope along with your request to:

AASECT
P.O. Box 238
Mount Vernon, IA 52314
http://www.aasect.org

In addition to all of the above, there is tremendous hope for the future development of medical therapy for female sexual dysfunction. Viagra, which is a drug that increases blood flow, has helped many thousands of men with erectile dysfunction. Early clinical studies of this drug with women identified as experiencing sexual dysfunction based in physiology show tremendous promise. Viagra, along with a multitude of other drugs that also enhance blood flow, are rapidly under development specifically for women and will soon need patients to sign up for clinical trials to determine whether or not they even work. While clinical trials are the only way in which we will advance medicine in this area, it's still important to retain your critical thinking and carefully review all the requirements and potential outcome of any medications before you join a clinical trial.

Over-the-counter herbal remedies, such as Yohimbine, are widely available and many individuals report successful enhancement of blood flow and reduced sexual dysfunction; but caution should always be taken when self-administering these drugs. Yes, herbal remedies are drugs—of the unregulated variety. As such, one should always have a firm understanding of the potential side effects before using these remedies. Yohimbine can cause a fast heartbeat, increased blood pressure, dizziness, headache, irritability, nervousness or restlessness, nausea and vomiting, skin flushing, sweating, and tremor. In addition, Yohimbine may make any number of other health conditions, such as kidney disease, worse. While most people may not experience any of these side effects, it is important to have an understanding that herbal remedies can be just as full of health risks as any prescribed medication.

Eight

Making a Decision

You've made it past basic anatomy class, learned how doctors can some-times present information to you in a way that influences your decisions, uncovered all your current treatment options, and discovered a few re-lated health issues along the way and, well, here you are. Are you ready to decide what to do next?

Making a treatment decision is simply not that easy. It wasn't for me, and perhaps it isn't easy for you either. There are many other things, be-yond your immediate health problems, that often end up influencing the final treatment decision. Although I wish it were that simple, **making a decision** is about a lot more than simply picking a treatment option.

Perhaps you've determined that your doctor is out-of-date and out to lunch with what he's told you about your uterine fibroids and treatment choices. Maybe you need to start looking for a new doctor. This is the chapter that will explain how to find a doctor you can really trust and work with on a solution to your health problems.

How do you know you're being told everything you need to know about a selected procedure and the doctor who will be performing it? Check out the section on informed consent (p. 158), which will give you some ideas on how to get the information you need from your physician.

In addition, this chapter also covers a few insurance issues, the influ-encing factors of friends, family members and co-workers, and a little bit about what MY choice was at the end of my journey for a solution.

Doctors

I'd **love** to be able to write that **all** doctors, *especially* gynecologists, are supportive, caring individuals who only have **your** best interests in mind when they take the necessary time to review with you **all** the medical options available to treat your uterine fibroids.

Unfortunately, the truth is not kind to either doctors or patients. Some doctors are simply not nice at all. Many have their own personal agendas. Some just don't seem to have enough time for you. Then again, maybe the problem is simply that it takes two people to really communicate and, for whatever reason, you and your doctor just can't find a way to have a meaningful and useful conversation. Rest assured that you are not alone in this regard. The individual who has *never* encountered a difficult communication session with a physician is rare today. After all, physicians are simply human beings with specialized training in medicine. I don't get along with every single person I encounter, and I bet you don't either. Medical professionals are not exceptional superhumans with super powers in the area of communication. They're just people.

Finding the Right Doctor

Choosing the right doctor can be an incredible task. Because there are so many interpersonal variables that play into a patient-physician relationship, there's no surefire method for hitting a home run with every doctor you pick. You may hear nothing but great things about a specific doctor and then find, much to your dismay, that the "great doctor" can't even look you in the eyes during a visit. Perhaps this bothers you. Perhaps it's simply a minor annoyance that can be overlooked. Everyone is different in what they require of their physicians *personally*—an excellent point to keep in mind when accepting referrals from the people you know.

It is, however, incredibly important that you feel comfortable enough to freely ask questions. In return, it's equally imperative to have a doctor offer information that makes sense to you. A physician should be open and willing to discuss with you the details of any medical exam or procedure and take the time necessary to ensure that you truly understand the information. If you have concerns, speak up. A good physician will listen. Positive, two-way communication can be a critical element in a patient-physician relationship. No matter how well qualified a doctor is—if you don't feel comfortable with the current line of communication, he's probably not the right physician for you.

If you find you simply can't communicate with your current doctor, *find a new one.* Keep looking until you find one that you *can* communicate with. End of story. Okay, okay. I know it's not that easy when you belong to a Health Maintenance Organization (HMO), live in a rural community, or rely on others to assist you in getting to a physician. But, *it's important.* Use common sense, listen to your intuition, and search until you find a doctor you can truly communicate with and whom you trust to provide you with all the medical options that are potential treatment choices for you to consider.

I know. Easier said than done. But, *at least try.* I did and I didn't. I regret that, in my case, I didn't try harder, but I just got tired of hearing the word *hysterectomy.* Don't make my mistake and wait until your fibroids are the size of a basketball or wreaking complete havoc with your life before you make the effort to find a doctor who meets your needs. Even if your fibroid symptoms are manageable right now, talk to your doctor about what your future options might be should your symptoms suddenly require treating the fibroids instead of treating only the symptoms. It's a good idea to open up this discussion early in the diagnosis and treatment of your fibroids so that you can determine whether or not the treatment options your physician has in mind for you are in line with your own thoughts on the subject.

In terms of competence and skill, it cannot be overstated that the more you know about a doctor before you ever set foot in his office, the better your chance of finding a physician who meets your needs the first time out.

State Medical Boards

Every physician is licensed to practice general medicine and surgery by a state board of medical examiners after passing a licensing examination. Whether you pick a doctor's name out of the phone book, your HMO book, or receive a referral from a physician referral service, friend, or family member, the next step (before you make an appointment!) is to verify their licensure and do a bit of a background check. To do this, contact your state medical board. (*See the State Medical Boards Appendix for a complete listing of all medical licensing agencies in the United States.*)

Every state in the United States has a medical board that oversees licensing of physicians and handles consumer (patient) complaints. As a rule of thumb, I **never** see a physician until I've checked out the status of the doctor's license. If you visit the website on the Internet for the state agency that licenses medical practitioners in your state, you can often obtain a great deal of information about a physician. For instance, the state of Tennessee (Tennessee Board of Medical Examiners) publicly discloses all the following about a physician:

- medical practice address
- languages spoken
- graduate/postgraduate medical/professional education and training
- specialty board certifications
- faculty appointments
- hospital staff privileges
- medical plan participation
- final disciplinary action
- criminal offenses
- liability claims

In addition, it allows a physician to provide optional information about community service awards or honors he has received. Publications in medical journals may also be detailed by the physician. Even with all this information available on the Internet, the Public Citizen's Health Research Group (HRG) conducted a 1999 *Survey of Doctor Disciplinary Information on State Medical Board websites* and gave Tennessee the grade of C for its online content. Only one state received an A grade for content—Maryland. So why did Tennessee receive a C? Because it doesn't provide any specific information about disciplinary action taken against a physician. Maryland not only provides this level of information; it also includes a narrative summary of any physician misconduct AND the full text of the state medical board's order for discipline.

Amazingly, this information is all free and available to the public by simply visiting the Maryland website or requesting the information through the mail or by telephone. Even though Tennessee is one of my favorite states for checking out doctors, the information they provide to the public would more comprehensively serve the public if it included more specific information about disciplinary action taken against physicians. Tennessee wasn't alone in receiving a poor grade from the Public Citizen's HRG though. Twenty-six states in all received a grade of C or lower.

If you live in California, the information provided by the Medical Board of California is minimal and includes only the doctor's name, basic licensing data, address, year of graduation, and medical school attended. If disciplinary action has been taken, that too is generally noted as part of the status code for the physician's license. However, getting details about that disciplinary action is like pulling teeth from a polar bear. The Medical Board of California certainly seems to be extremely protective of the information it acquires on physicians practicing medicine in that state. California is not alone in this regard, though. Many other states are also extremely protective of their physicians, and this can make a background check rather difficult. Every state reporting agency is different because every state sets its own laws regarding the licensing and public disclosure of information on a medical licensee to the general public. It's truly unfortunate that this information is not uniformly available to consumers on a national basis.

Perhaps checking on a doctor's medical license and background may seem a bit silly to some of you. You trust your doctor because he's the same one you've been seeing for years. And, of course a doctor wouldn't be in an office taking patients if he weren't properly licensed, right? Wrong. Twice in the last year alone I came across doctors identified in my husband's HMO doctor directory who were, in fact, no longer licensed to practice medicine in the state of California. Both still had offices, and a nurse-practitioner was seeing patients while new physicians were being sought to fill the previous physicians' slots. One of the doctors was someone my teenage daughter had seen previously, but suddenly she couldn't get past the nurse-practitioner to see the doctor to save her soul. I became a bit suspicious and decided to check the medical licensing for the physician on the Internet. Boy, was I surprised to find that the doctor had chosen not to renew her license! You'd think the medical staff would tell you that when you book an appointment, wouldn't you? But, they didn't.

You just never know. It can be very important to check.

Take, for instance, my own personal experience with Dr. Vicki Hufnagel as I was researching female reconstructive surgery (FRS) years ago.

A Word about State Medical Boards

State medical boards can often be bureaucratic nightmares to retrieve any information from at all. As a medical consumer, I've often wondered about their true worth in serving me and protecting me from physicians who do real harm.

In several states, when checking on physician records, I've encountered phone transfer after phone transfer after phone transfer. Lots of dead ends and not an answer in sight to my questions. Rude responses from clerical staff that aren't legally able to answer any question over the telephone. Typical suggestions are to "submit it in writing" or "fax your question" with little to no understanding from the party on the other end how hard it was to even pick up the phone and call in the first place. On top of that, even when you do "submit it in writing" they can take their precious sweet time in responding.

It's discouraging at best, and definitely gives the impression that they are not there to serve you, the medical consumer.

All this can make it a real pain to get an answer to a simple question or to file a complaint. Nonetheless, they ARE the agency that oversees licensing of physicians and handling of consumer complaints. When you contact your state medical board, muster up an extra dose of patience and perseverance and hang in there until you get your questions answered and/or your complaint fully registered.

On average, 1,600 physicians' licenses are revoked annually in the United States. So, even with all the bureaucratic hoops one must jump through to get an answer or file a complaint, the medical boards in this country MUST be doing something about the complaints they receive. Sometimes, however, it just takes longer than any of us ever anticipate to get the action we would like to see occur immediately.

This physician was about to lose her license in the state of California and there I was, getting in line for surgery with her! Checking with the state medical board on her licensure status stopped me cold.

Board Certification

Beyond a doctor's training in general medicine, training in certain specialties can take an additional two to ten years. Board certification of that additional training can be an important sign of a physician's additional education and experience beyond his residency training. It can also demonstrate a physician's desire to continue learning about his chosen specialty field of medicine (like gynecology or radiology or laparoscopy).

In order to be board certified, a physician must complete certain requirements in addition to obtaining a medical degree and completing a residency program. All specialty medical boards are different, but requirements a physician must meet for certification might include:

- assessment of individual performance and competence from the residency training director of the hospital where the doctor practiced
- unrestricted licensing to practice medicine
- experience in a full-time practice in the specialty prior to examination for board certification, usually at least two years following training
- passage of a written examination given by the specialty board
- passage of an oral examination given by senior board certified members in that field

Doctors who pass the exams and additional requirements are given the status of Diplomate and are board certified as specialists. It would stand to reason that doctors who make this effort of acquiring board certification in their medical specialty would represent physicians who have stronger skills and a desire to meet certain standards of practice. Sometimes this isn't the case. But, as a benchmark of skills acquired, this is at least a notch above the medical degree and residency training that all doctors go through.

Keep in mind that not all physicians are board certified. To determine whether or not your selected physician has any board certifications, check with the American Board of Medical Specialties (ABMS) (http://www.certifieddoctor.org/); or, you can simply ask your doctor. If your doctor is NOT board certified, you should definitely ask why not and listen very carefully to the response you receive. He may be working on acquiring board certification, he may have chosen not to bother with board certification, or he may have not passed board certification. You'll never know unless you ask.

Certificate of Added Qualification (CAQ)

In addition to board certification, interventional radiologists can also work for and acquire a Certificate of Added Qualification (CAQ) granted by the American Board of Radiology. To earn this added certification, an interventional radiologist must successfully complete one year of fellowship training (after residency) in a Vascular and Interventional program accredited by the Accreditation Council for Graduate Medical Education. He must also have completed one year of practice or additional approved training in Vascular and Interventional Radiology.

To qualify for the oral exam, the interventional radiologist must show proof of having completed at least 500 cases that show diverse experience in vascular and nonvascular interventions.

If you are considering UAE as a treatment option, looking for an interventional radiologist who has earned this CAQ can give you some added assurance that the physician has seriously sought out and acquired additional training and validation of his skills through a formal course of review and examination.

Background Check

An additional way to obtain background information on your selected physician is to contact the American Medical Association at (312) 464-5199. By telephone, you can get information on more than seven hundred thousand doctors practicing in the United States. For around $60 (call for current prices), you can write and receive profiles on as many as five doctors, including address, age, birthplace, education, specialties, board certifications, and disciplinary actions. Send the names of up to five doctors and a check to:

AMA, Department of Data Services
515 N. State St.
Chicago, IL 60610

Don't forget to include your name and the address at which you wish to receive the report.

By computer, the AMA website (http://www.ama-assn.org/) contains some, but not all, of the same information, including a doctor finder, hospital finder, and medical group practice finder.

Medi-Net

For an even MORE complete background check on your selected physician, you may want to contact Medi-Net, a private reporting firm located in Carlsbad, California at (888) 275-6334. The price for a Medi-Net report is extremely reasonable—approximately $15 for the first doctor and about $5 for each additional doctor. (Call for current prices.) Medi-Net can provide you with a printout containing the following information:

- medical school and year of graduation
- residency training, including the name of the hospital, length of time spent training there, and any specialized training received
- American Board of Medical Specialties Certifications
- states in which the physician is currently licensed, as well as historical licensure data across **all** states
- records of sanctions or disciplinary actions taken against a physician's license, if any, from **all** states
- If a specified doctor is disciplined within a year of your report request, Medi-Net will send you notification for free.

Before paying for this information, however, it's still a good idea to check with your own state medical board, because most of the above information may be available through them for free. Not all state medical boards offer this level of detailed information, though, and when in doubt, Medi-Net provides comprehensive information about a physician's medical practice background from every state.

Special Procedures: Endoscopic Surgery (Laparoscopy/Hysteroscopy)

Laparoscopy and hysteroscopy are two procedures that fall under the specialty category of endoscopy. With endoscopy, special equipment is used to go inside the uterus or abdomen to visualize the interior of a

woman's body and to perform procedures such as laparoscopic myomectomy, hysteroscopic myomectomy, or laparoscopically assisted hysterectomy. All doctors certified in obstetrics and gynecology are trained to use
this equipment. That does **not** mean, however, that they are all equally
skilled at using this equipment.

The Accreditation Council for Gynecologic Endoscopy (ACGE) was set
up to determine standards in operative endoscopic procedures performed
by gynecologists. Surgeons who consider themselves advanced operators
in endoscopic surgery and demonstrate sufficient case documentation
may become certified through the ACGE. For more information on locating doctors who've demonstrated to a review board of peers that they've
performed a high number of endoscopy procedures, contact the ACGE at:

Accreditation Council for Gynecologic Endoscopy
P.O. Box 610
Downey, CA 90241-0610
Phone: (562) 946-4435
http://www.aagl.com/acgel.htm

A Few Additional Items to Check

Once you've located a doctor who meets your medical competence and
skill requirements, there are a few more things that can be checked that
will give you a much bigger picture of his overall ability to meet your
medical needs. Because communication can be a huge obstacle in patient-
physician relationships, find out whether or not the physician is willing
to take some time to chat with you before scheduling a formal visit. Many
doctors understand how hard it is to "shop" for a physician. When given
the opportunity, take the time to meet with him. The following is a starter
list of questions that you can use in learning more about the physician
and his practice. *Even though you may have already obtained this information through another source, it is still a good idea to ask the questions
and get a conversation going with the physician to determine how well the
two of you communicate.*

1. Ask the doctor for the names of hospitals where he has admitting
   privileges. If the doctor doesn't have hospital admitting privileges, ask
   why not.

2. Does the physician have associates, and would you feel comfortable being treated by them if your doctor is not available?
3. Does the doctor use well-trained staff, such as registered nurses and physician assistants? Are there enough of them? Are they friendly?
4. Does the doctor seem friendly and knowledgeable?
5. Are you comfortable and confident with the doctor? (*Do you feel that you can really have a conversation and discuss EVERYTHING with this doctor, or does he make you want to "clam up"?*)
6. Is the office clean and well organized? (*An unorganized office can be a sign of poor management and disorganized record keeping.*)

Asking direct questions, as with the first question listed above, when you're in the early stages of trying to develop a new patient-physician relationship may seem like a difficult and delicate task. Don't worry if you find yourself struggling to get the words out. If you need to, simply write out each of your questions and take a notepad with you to write down the answers. Many doctors have come to expect and sincerely appreciate patients who come to them with a written list of questions and concerns.

With uterine fibroids, concerns you may have about care and treatment options are also extremely important—especially in an initial contact with a new physician. You can find out very early if this is a physician you can work with by simply asking for more information on his treatment perspective of uterine fibroids.

If you've been seeing a physician for some time and he suddenly tells you that you need a hysterectomy but doesn't present any other treatment options, you need to find out why. Remember, in most cases uterine fibroids are not life threatening and any treatment at all is considered an *elective choice* that you simply make—not a choice that is truly required. Take the time to gather the information you need before you make a decision or schedule surgery. In fact, **never** schedule elective surgery for any medical condition on the same day that it is suggested to you by a physician. Go home, think about it, gather more information, and *get a second opinion.*

Whether the physician is one you've known for a long time or a new one you're attempting to establish a relationship with, it's important to find out what procedures the physician has, in fact, performed for the treatment of uterine fibroids. What were some of the more difficult cases the physician has handled and whom did he confer with about those cases? Also, what referrals were made to other physicians when his own skills were not appropriate for the patient's medical situation or preferred treatment option?

For instance, if you are interested in uterine artery embolization as a treatment option, has the doctor ever referred anyone for this procedure? If so, what was the name of the referred interventional radiologist? If you are considering myomectomy, how many has the doctor performed and what were some of the complications encountered? Does myolysis interest you? Try to find out what the doctor thinks about it as a treatment option *before* you schedule an appointment. Is the doctor certified in endoscopy and/or comfortable with performing endoscopy? If not, this could very well be the primary reason for the doctor recommending an abdominal incision instead of using laparoscopy for myomectomy or hysterectomy.

All in all, it may be a good idea to find out just what treatment options *might* be offered to you before you ever make an appointment. In most cases, if the physician has a predisposition to performing a lot of hysterectomies, you are very likely to figure it out by the answers he gives you to alternative treatment option questions.

If the responses to any of your questions are hostile or evasive, trust your instincts and reevaluate everything you know about the physician. Hostility and evasiveness are not usually good signs. It's probably a clear indication of the type of treatment you will receive as a patient. So, is this really the physician for you?

File a Complaint

Okay. So you did all the appropriate checks and found the doctor you're seeing *is* licensed, legit, and maybe even board certified. You thought you asked all the right questions "up front" and were even satisfied with the answers you received. Nonetheless, you discover that the doctor is a day late and a dollar short in terms of his bedside manner and quality of care and, just maybe, incredibly inept in his overall medical skills. Perhaps you had a rough time with the doctor during an examination and don't ever want to return to him again. Well, DON'T! Listen to your instincts and find another doctor.

If you believe that what your doctor has done to you is wrong or indicative of medical negligence or malpractice, *please,* oh *please* file a

Gynecologists Who Refer Patients for Uterine Artery Embolization

Some gynecologists are now advertising that they refer patients for uterine artery embolization (UAE) when, in fact, they do not. In order to protect yourself from this kind of unscrupulous medical behavior, I recommend the following questions be asked of the doctor when scheduling your first appointment:

1. How many women have you referred for UAE?
2. How many women that you referred actually chose UAE?
3. What is the name of the interventional radiologist whom you've used for referral?

Be sure to get the name of the hospital and the phone number of the interventional radiologist from the gynecologist (or a staff person) and then CALL the interventional radiologist to verify the information that was given to you. Find out what, exactly, the experience has been of the interventional radiologist with the specific gynecologist. You need to know what kind of support and communication you can expect from both parties should you choose to proceed with uterine artery embolization. If you find that the interventional radiologist has never even heard your gynecologist's name previously and hasn't received any referrals from him, you might find this a good time to ask for a referral to a gynecologist whom the interventional radiologist DOES know.

In checking on several prominent gynecologists who indicated (online or in advertising) that they referred patients for UAE, I discovered that reality could be a very ugly thing. Once women make appointments and meet with the gynecologist, their particular circumstances seem to exclude them from being good candidates for UAE. Further checking told me that those very gynecologists NEVER actually referred a single woman for UAE. But it makes good advertising copy to say that they do, doesn't it?

Of course, not every woman with uterine fibroids IS a good candidate for UAE. But to ensure that you will receive fair and even representation of your options, it is a good idea to follow through on the suggestions presented in this chapter.

If your current gynecologist or a gynecologist you are attempting to establish a patient-physician relationship with has NEVER referred a woman for UAE but expresses to you that he would be willing to consider such a referral, ask him the name of the interventional radiologist that he would use for referral. Ask him if he has actually spoken to the specific interventional radiologist yet to determine, collaboratively, what patient selection criteria should be followed for referral.

Communication between the gynecologist and the interventional radiologist must be set in motion BEFORE your first appointment (to see a new gynecologist) or the likelihood that you will be wasting your time and money is very high.

complaint with your state medical board! You don't have to hire an attorney or file a lawsuit to file a complaint and, quite possibly, have actions sanctioned against a physician. You simply need to fill out a few forms and send them in. That's it. Medical negligence or malpractice is a very serious charge against a physician. Even so, the filing of a complaint may be critical to the health and welfare of that physician's future patients.

The only way for you and me to "weed out" the physicians who don't deserve a medical license is to be proactive in our selection of physicians and filing of complaints, when necessary. Not everyone who makes it through medical school and receives her/his license deserves to be practicing medicine. We simply **must** complain about incompetent medical care to the proper authorities—instead of just walking away and whining about it.

In the United States there are eight times as many instances of negligence as there are claims for compensation. In general, instead of dealing with the paperwork hassles of filing a complaint, most people simply walk away and allow the physician to continue to do harm to others. Perhaps if we all did our part in reporting bad medical practitioners, we would help protect one another and, in the end, get rid of doctors who don't deserve to be doctors.

Informed Consent

In the medical world (and legal world), the concept of *informed consent* relates to a patient's receipt of enough specific and relevant information to then allow that patient to make an informed decision about treatment and consent to medical care. It is the right of every individual considering any medical procedure in the United States to receive appropriate information that would allow him or her to then give the caregiver *informed consent* to proceed with treatment.

Generally speaking, informed consent lays down a road map for the kind of information that a physician or medical institution is required to tell a patient about a proposed medical procedure. Admission forms that are signed by anyone entering a hospital in the United States could be considered one type of informed consent. Informed consent for an elective medical procedure should include, at a minimum, the following:

> ➤ identification of the physician/surgeon performing the procedure
> ➤ the patient's present condition
> ➤ the purpose of the proposed procedure
> ➤ the risks involved in the procedure
> ➤ the treatment alternatives INCLUDING the risks of the alternatives (if nontreatment is an option, the risk of that as well)

Where treatment options for uterine fibroids are concerned, there is a major problem with the concept of informed consent. This problem has its foundation in something often referred to as the *Standard of Care*. If a specific treatment for a specific disease has been identified by the medical community as the "standard" treatment of care, then any and all other treatment options do not *have* to be presented to the patient as a possible option. Good physicians will, of course, communicate information about all known treatment options to their patients—but they aren't, necessarily, required to do so. The *standard of care* for symptomatic uterine fibroids in women who do not desire fertility is currently identified by the American College of Obstetricians and Gynecologists as hysterectomy. Consequently, in forty-seven out of fifty states a physician is not *required* to share information regarding any other treatment option for uterine fibroids. The remaining three states—California, Texas, and New York—have state legislation that requires a physician to more thoroughly identify and explain a patient's medical situation and her options specifically in cases involving hysterectomy as a treatment option. New York's laws on this issue are the most comprehensive anywhere in the United

States and the New York Department of Health publishes a public information booklet that is distributed to all patients who've received the recommendation for a hysterectomy.

It's truly unfortunate that laws regulating the communication flow from physicians to patients have to be voted into place, and I wish I could say that they are unnecessary adjuncts to the fundamental concept of informed consent. Medical literature clearly shows, however, that unnecessary and inappropriately recommended hysterectomies are being performed at far too high a rate. One *Journal of Public Health* study revealed that, depending upon the race of the patient, 4 to 9 percent of the women who underwent hysterectomy as identified on hospital discharge records for the diagnosis of uterine fibroids, showed no disease whatsoever on the pathology reports. Another study showed the rate as high as 14 percent (14 percent of 600,000 hysterectomies = 84,000 unnecessary procedures).

In the Appendix, you'll find a sample form of an Informed Consent document for Total Abdominal Hysterectomy. This document contains the kind of information necessary to adequately identify the risks involved with this procedure. Unfortunately, I've never seen an informed consent document for any medical procedure that contains the level of detail provided in this sample. Nor have I seen a form such as this that requires initials for specific consent of individual items.

There is a great deal of controversy surrounding informed consent. Most consent forms are extremely brief, typically presented with at least some text on the form so small you'd need a magnifying glass to read it and without a request for signatures or initials throughout the document that might indicate the individual actually read each and every portion of the form. Some doctors think that a detailed form, such as this sample, should also contain a listing of the benefits that might be obtained from a medical procedure so as to bring balance to the risks AND benefits of the surgery. Of course, when the doctor indicates the purpose of the proposed procedure, there is ample opportunity to list all the benefits of the procedure to the patient.

Once informed consent has been given and agreed to by both the physician and the patient, the physician may NOT exceed the scope of the consent except when reasonable actions must be taken to save the life of the patient due to unexpected events during surgery. This is an important point to make because far too often a gynecologist will use the

ACOG (Standard of Care) guidelines for hysterectomy (when uterine fibroids are present) to proceed with removal of the uterus, ovaries, and the cervix—even when there were prior conversations and verbal consent was given by the patient to removal of ONLY uterine fibroids. This is not acceptable to me, and it shouldn't be to you either. "Lifesaving measures" need to be indicated on the form and indicated during the procedure before a physician has a right to wander off the path of what was agreed upon by performing a hysterectomy instead of myomectomy.

This is an extremely gray area of what can or cannot be done by a physician when a woman is under anesthesia. It is the primary reason why many women do not trust gynecologists who say they will "try" to do a myomectomy. Too often, a woman wakes up after myomectomy surgery to discover her physician performed a hysterectomy instead. Women talk about these incidents when they occur. Some of us have heard a story or two that rattles us and makes it difficult for us to simply trust the words coming out of a physician's mouth. The sheer quantity of email that I receive on this topic from women who trusted their doctors completely to perform a myomectomy and ended up with a total pelvic clean out (TAH/BSO) instead makes me sad, mad, and thoroughly disgusted. We must simply take control over our own bodies and our future health as much as possible and insist upon appropriate informed consent information prior to agreeing to any medical procedure.

It's appalling to me how many women undergo hysterectomy without adequate information on what, exactly, is going to occur during surgery. What is going to be removed? If the doctor is unsure, what are the guidelines that will be followed in removing the uterus, ovaries, or cervix? Additionally appalling is the number of women who never had discussions with their doctors about the aftereffects of the surgery. What are the potential outcomes? What could, possibly, go wrong?

Let's not forget to mention the frequently forgotten issue of hormone replacement therapy. Whether the ovaries are being removed or not, the potential for ovarian failure post-hysterectomy is incredibly high and often occurs within five years of the hysterectomy. It seems to me that a discussion regarding the potential need for hormone replacement therapy should be right up front in any discussion of hysterectomy and outcome. But, often, it's never mentioned until the woman begins asking questions post-hysterectomy due to problems she is experiencing that she just can't figure out.

First and foremost, before you ever get to the hysterectomy, did your doctor tell you anything at all about the other treatment choices available for uterine fibroids? This is one of the five critical items that make up informed consent.

Not a single physician recommending hysterectomy in my fourteen years of refusing surgery and allowing the fibroids to continue to grow ever discussed ANY of the issues listed above. Even when I attempted to discuss myomectomy with several different doctors, it was immediately dismissed as not an option for me. No other options were ever even presented or discussed. In addition, surgical outcomes and hormone replacement therapy were never mentioned. Postprocedure side effects were not issues up for discussion as, of course, those things wouldn't happen to me.

How do doctors get away with this?

Through inaction, we give doctors permission to continue to:

- *make limited recommendations (i.e., hysterectomy-only option)*
- *perform potentially unnecessary procedures*
- *retain control over the future health of our bodies*

Ultimately, WE are the bearers of the consequences of our inaction and ignorance of medical procedures. WE are the ones who must live with the surgical outcome, good or bad.

When do most patients actually see an informed consent document for a medical procedure? Most of us are handed a form to sign only minutes before a procedure is to be performed. This is something that is far too often *standard operating procedure* for physicians and hospitals. It is unreasonable to expect any patient to read the fine details of these forms and understand what, precisely, she is signing when she consents to a procedure under those circumstances. Why can't doctors and hospitals get a form to a patient at least three business days in advance? Certainly medical procedures done to our bodies are as important as purchasing a vacuum cleaner at home (with three days to change your mind on most major contracts in most states)! But only minutes before a procedure or on the same day as checking into the hospital? Give me a break! Although many a doctor may disagree with me, I personally believe that true informed consent does not occur on the day of the procedure. Consent for a surgical procedure obtained the day of the procedure or shortly before the procedure constitutes informed consent submitted to under duress.

So, if you can get informed consent documentation to read and review in advance of a procedure, by all means do so. At least ask your doctor for this information—perhaps you'll be pleasantly surprised to find out you have a progressive doctor with the details already put together in a handy-dandy form for you to take home and share with your family. It couldn't hurt to at least ask.

Perhaps you live in one of the forty-seven states without informed consent laws that relate specifically to hysterectomy. Wouldn't you prefer to be assured that when you visit your gynecologist and are given the hysterectomy-indicated song and dance for your fibroids the physician be obligated to inform you of 1) other treatment options, 2) potential surgical outcomes, and 3) potential need for hormone replacement therapy? If so, take the time to learn more about this issue of informed consent and get involved in changing the laws to more positively reflect the needs of the women in your community.

There is a great deal of information about informed consent on the Internet and many websites address this issue with ideas on how you can better protect yourself. They also offer advice on how to get involved with changing your own state's laws. While I was searching for more information on this topic, I came across many websites written specifically for physicians to help them gain an understanding of how to better protect themselves against patient lawsuits. These websites gave me a great deal of insight into how doctors are protecting themselves. What I want to know is **How are we, as patients, protecting ourselves?**

Insurance

The number-one question that seems to get asked over and over again regarding medical insurance is NOT how to find the best insurance plan or provider, but rather:

How do you overturn a denial for treatment?

Denial for treatments requiring preauthorization is occurring on a scale that can only be described as *phenomenal*. Any procedure offered that doesn't result in a "definitive" outcome for the treatment of uterine fibroids is tagged as being less than desirable by insurance providers. There is a definite push by insurance providers for women to choose only the hysterectomy option—regardless of the man hours lost due to the recovery period of a hysterectomy (6-8 weeks); regardless of the known post-hysterectomy complications that might result in additional, long-term care; regardless of a woman's desire to keep her uterus.

Although many insurance providers would prefer that a woman making a treatment choice for fibroids choose hysterectomy, treatment of uterine fibroids is an *elective choice* that an individual makes for the treatment of a *benign* disease. As such, many insurance plans choose to deny treatment coverage unless a patient's medical record clearly shows symptomatic fibroids and an adequate effort at treating symptoms first—even when the recommendation is hysterectomy.

I know. You're thinking that because there are so many hysterectomies performed in the United States each year that surely women who choose hysterectomy never encounter a problem with insurance coverage. Unfortunately, they do. Not all—but some do. This denial of coverage is usually for one of many possible reasons. Take your pick from the list below or make one up from your own experience with insurance providers:

1. An insurance company/reviewer might deny coverage because the medical chart doesn't adequately indicate the need for the procedure. It is determined the procedure is *not medically necessary*.
2. An insurance company/reviewer might deny all major medical procedures the first time they are requested. Without any real reasoning.
3. An insurance company might save money if they deny coverage because some patients retreat and end up not undergoing any procedure.
4. An insurance company can keep and invest their capital a little longer and earn more money from it if they deny coverage for a procedure and delay a claim.
5. An insurance company might believe they are protecting their plan participant (you) from an investigational/experimental procedure with unproven outcome when they deny coverage.

What can you do if you are denied coverage for your chosen procedure? Well, you can pay cash out of your own pocket. This isn't, however, a very practical suggestion for most of us. We buy medical insurance to protect us from large out-of-pocket medical expenses precisely because we couldn't possibly afford to pay for these big-ticket items all at once with cash when we encounter them. Large medical bills for surgical treatment are economic disasters for most families. Besides, we paid for medical insurance coverage. Don't we have a right to expect it to be there when we need it?

So, what *can* you do? If you are currently looking at an insurance denial letter and believe your case should have been approved, then the following steps and information may help you successfully appeal your case.

1. Educate yourself about your condition and ALL your options. Is the procedure your doctor recommended REALLY the best one for you and your condition?

2. Request a copy of your insurance plan's policies and read everything you can about the procedures that are covered. If you are requesting a specific procedure like hysterectomy, myomectomy, or uterine artery embolization, you may have to specifically call and request the policy statement the plan has that details the specifics of coverage for those procedures. Not all plan booklets go into this detail.

3. Carefully document everything. Take notes of every phone conversation you have with your insurance company. (This will come in handy later if you need to file a lawsuit based on any medical need that wasn't addressed appropriately by your insurance company. I hope this won't happen—but you never know.)

4. Request a copy of your medical records from your physician. Compare your chart against what the insurance company outlines as requirements to approve the procedure. Work with your physician to ensure that all requirements are met. This may include attempts at treating the symptoms, undergoing appropriate diagnostic tests to confirm your uterine fibroids and rule out other disease and finally, medically documenting everything in an organized manner that would lend itself to leading up to the referred procedure. Your physician needs to create a very clean, very clear road map on your medical chart that sincerely indicates a strong need for the desired procedure and *only the desired procedure*. All other potential procedures need to be ruled out with reasons stated as to why. If this isn't done, a reviewer may well return the request with a recommendation for some other procedure or medical treatment instead.

5. Appeal every denial. In doing so, write simply and make your letters as short as possible. Do not, however, leave out important details surrounding your case. Write a personal plea detailing your health history as it relates to your current condition. Make the letter as brief as possible (no rambling), but include the following:

➤ Explain why you want and need the procedure you've requested. How are your symptoms impacting your Quality of Life?

➤ Explain why each and every other treatment option is an inappropriate choice for you. For instance, if you are attempting to get uterine artery embolization approved, specifically state why "watchful waiting," "medical therapy" (progestin/oral contraceptives), myomectomy, hysterectomy, endometrial ablation, etc., are not valid approaches to your situation.

➤ Identify what you have done, over time, to try to live with or resolve your health symptoms from fibroids.

➤ If your symptoms include abnormal bleeding, the following are a few of the items that reviewers look for and expect to see addressed by either you or your physician in your appeal letter:

✓ Have you tried medical therapy (oral contraceptives/progestin) in an attempt to regulate your menstrual cycle/bleeding? If so, what was the outcome?

✓ Have you undergone an endometrial biopsy to rule out hyperplasia or endometrial cancer?

✓ Are you anemic? If so, have you been treated with iron? What were the results?

NOTE: If your blood tests do not show that you are anemic but at the same time you are passing blood clots during your period and you're tired all the time, is it possible that blood tests are being drawn during a time when you are not menstruating? Most women attempt to schedule gynecological exams when they are not bleeding. A blood test administered during the peak of passing blood clots each month might provide you with different results that do show anemia.

✓ Have you had a transvaginal ultrasound and/or MRI within the last six months?

✓ What are the size and location of your fibroids?

> **NOTE:** Size and location are critical factors that should be playing a role in your choice of treatment. For example, if your fibroids are submucosal and you are seeking UAE, would hysteroscopic resection of the fibroid be a better option? If not, why not? If your fibroids are subserosal and you are seeking UAE, would laparoscopic myomectomy be a better option? If not, why not? Consider all the potential treatment options and determine viability, risk, and outcome and present a logical justification for your treatment choice.

6. Ask your gynecologist to write a supportive letter verifying the details of your letter and detailing your current medical condition, what therapies have been tried, what failed, and what his professional opinion is regarding the need for the treatment desired. This is a critical piece of your appeal and can not and should not be overlooked no matter which treatment option you desire.

7. If you are seeking approval for UAE, ask your interventional radiologist to write a supportive letter verifying your need for the procedure and the anticipated outcome. It may also be important to include additional information that technically details the procedure and identifies known outcome from current studies. Include copies of published medical reports and/or a detailed bibliography of peer-reviewed documentation. The information that either you or your interventional radiologist provides with your appeal should show the length of time the procedure has been around, the clinical studies or trials that have been completed, and the overall documented outcome of the procedure you are requesting.

➤ Some procedures haven't been around very long and as such are classified as investigational or experimental. Uterine artery embolization, myolyis, and even laparoscopic myomectomy are all considered "investigational" by many insurance companies. Even the American College of Obstetricians and Gynecologists has gone on record as saying the ". . . benefit of laparoscopic removal of leiomyomata has not been established . . ." Just because a procedure is deemed investigational by a company does not, however, mean that it won't be covered or paid for by your insurance provider. Do not give up simply because the insurance company denied you coverage based on an investigational or experimental status of the procedure.

8. Before mailing, photocopy everything in the packet. Keep one set for your own file and then make any number of additional copies for legislative representatives of your choice and the insurance regulatory body that oversees insurance providers within your state (see steps 9 and 10, below). Mail within the time frame allocated to you for an appeal (this varies by state and by provider) and send it all certified mail with return receipt.

> **NOTE:** If this is your FINAL appeal option, you may want to seek legal representation to guide you through this process. Although not entirely necessary, establishing a relationship with an attorney in your final phase of appeal can help you to move forward much quicker with civil litigation should you, once again, be denied coverage for treatment.

9. If you consider the denial you received unjustified and communication from your insurance provider entirely inappropriate, you may want to consider the involvement of your legislative representatives. Names, addresses, and phone numbers for all current legislative representatives are available online at the **Patient Advocacy (http://www.patientadvocacy.org)** website and also published in the booklet entitled *U.S. Congress Handbook—State Edition.* This booklet is published for each new Congress by the National Committee to Preserve Social Security and Medicare and is available free of charge by calling 1(800) 966-1935.

   Once you identify who you want to involve in your case, telephone their office(s) and ask specifically for the name of the person handling health insurance or HMO issues within the representative's office for your state. Obtain a name, telephone number, and email address, and then call or contact the individual personally, if possible. At a minimum, direct all correspondence to your chosen representative with an **ATTENTION:** to the person you've identified as handling health issues.

NOTE: In order for someone to act on your behalf, all correspondence to legislative representatives and/or patient advocates requesting action or involvement on their part regarding your personal health issues **must** include a letter authorizing them to access your medical records and speak for you.

10. Finally, it may also be appropriate to submit your appeal, along with a letter of explanation and a formal complaint, to the medical insurance regulatory body for your state. A complete list of contact information for each state is available by visiting the website for the National Association of Insurance Commissioners at **http://www.naic. org** or by writing or calling them and requesting this information for your state.

   National Association of Insurance Commissioners
   120 W. 12th Street, Suite 1100
   Kansas City, MO 64105
   (816) 842-3600 or (816) 374-7175

   Although state insurance regulatory bodies cannot FORCE your insurance provider to approve your treatment choice, they can be influential and have an impact.

No matter how angry and frustrated you may get, always be polite and courteous to your insurance representatives. I'm not saying you should let someone railroad you and walk all over you. Be firm but polite. (*In my case, I found that a simple plea of desperation and true need was met with a sympathetic ear and a fast response for approval. Of course, I had to get past the intake telephone personnel first. It took me several phone calls and no action on the part of my insurance company before I finally just asked the intake person if I could speak to a reviewer of claims. Then, I politely asked the reviewer why my request for approval was taking so long when I was in so much need. My claim was approved within 24 hours from that phone conversation.*) Never give up, no matter what. I know that not everyone is going to be so lucky as to get a sympathetic reviewer who quickly turns a denial into an approval. Try not to be intimidated by your insurance company and hang in there, appealing each denial.

If all this sounds like a lot of work, you're right. It is. There are many patient advocates who will work with you to help you through this process. Some will do so for free—some charge a fee. Many can be found on the Internet, but they are sometimes also listed in your telephone directory. Hang in there and do your best to fight for what is rightfully your medical decision to make—not your insurance provider's.

Friends, Family, and Co-workers

Friends, family members, and co-workers can be an incredibly valuable source of information and support as you attempt to sort out the medical details of your own specific medical condition and the treatment options available to you. They rally to your aid, offer you wisdom and advice in the choices they made, help you with research and locating appropriate doctors, and, all in all, show an outstanding level of love and kindness to you that you may have never known existed before. You may even, quite suddenly, find yourself privy to the most intimate details of the lives of any or all these people. When you open yourself up and allow people to know that you have uterine fibroids, you will be amazed at what tumbles out of their hearts as well as their mouths. Because so many women experience symptomatic uterine fibroids, it's a sure bet that nearly everyone knows someone who has had to deal with them.

Can this be a bad thing? Maybe. Not necessarily, though. It *can* bring about closeness with key individuals in your life that you never experienced before. It *can* give you insight into how someone else experienced and dealt with her uterine fibroids. More than anything else, it *can* show you how much you are loved and cared for by others.

Then again, it can just as easily be a thorn in your side. Justifying all statements to you as well intentioned and "*only looking out for your best interests,*" it's incredible what thoughtless people will say. You may find people who climb out of the woodwork just to register their two cents—completely unsolicited. They just might even drive you nuts asking questions about the specifics of your condition and put your ideas, principles, and treatment choice to the test! They may even believe that they have the right to question the very core of who you are and why you made such a (dumb) decision (in terms of your treatment choice).

First rule of thumb for dealing with these people? Don't share anything that makes you uncomfortable. No one really needs to know the specific details of your medical condition or treatment choice except you. My favorite line became:

"I'm not really comfortable talking about this. Do you mind if we don't discuss it anymore?"

It worked for me. It might work for you. Of course, you can always come up with your own standard line that changes the discussion topic. Sometimes, however, the only thing you can do is simply walk away from the discussion. Whatever you do, try to remember that these people think they are *helping* you. Leave room in your heart for the *possibility* that they truly are well intentioned. Then move on to talking about something else!

Regardless of the advice, information, and support you receive, friends, family members, and co-workers cannot tell you with any certainty what YOUR specific outcome will be with YOUR treatment choice. Everyone is different. Time and medical advances constantly alter the procedures that are available as well as the current thought processes that guide doctors in helping to inform you of what YOUR options are for treatment. It's important to keep this in mind as you go about discussing and seeking firsthand information from the friends, family members, and co-workers who so generously and freely share their thoughts and experiences with you.

My Choice

On November 2, 1998, I underwent uterine artery embolization (UAE), performed by Dr. Scott Goodwin at the University of California at Los Angeles Medical Center. It was not an easy decision. Years and years of the **Ignore the Fibroids** route. A few years of the **Treat the Symptoms** route. And, finally, the **Clinical Research** route. I did not want a hysterectomy. Not a single doctor recommended myomectomy or would agree to perform one when questioned about it as an option. Along the way, doctors made all the following statements to me:

- *Mrs. Dionne—you have a fibroid tumor. It's nothing, really. No need to worry. These things generally resolve themselves one way or another.*
- *Okay. It's time. It has to come out now.*

- *But, Mrs. Dionne, you've already had your children. Why would you want to keep your uterus?* (Stated more times by more doctors than I can possibly count.)
- *Why would you want to risk the possibility of cancerous fibroids?*
- *The uterus has no purpose except to bear children.*
- *A myomectomy is too risky. You could lose a lot of blood and even die. Would you really want to do that to your family?*
- *Read this.* (The doctor hands me a cartoon booklet created by a pharmaceutical manufacturer of hormone replacement therapy—synthetic progesterone and estrogen.) *It will set your mind at ease about the hysterectomy I'm going to schedule for you.* This doctor took the cake. Even though I told him that I did NOT want a hysterectomy, he scheduled it anyway *without my consent. I discovered this fact when the hospital called for preadmission information.* Needless to say, I canceled the scheduled surgery. The gynecologist then proceeded to call and pester me, trying desperately to convince me to undergo surgery, for quite some time.
- *Now take this video home and watch it. These women all felt so much better after their hysterectomy.* (I watched the video. It, too, was created by a pharmaceutical manufacturer of hormone replacement therapy and consisted of four testimonials. The women said nothing about hysterectomy. The whole video was a sales job on how hormone replacement therapy made their lives better.)
- *Sex is no reason to keep your uterus. Your uterus can't feel anything during sex. Sex for women is purely clitoral.*

I could go on. Every doctor had his or her say. In addition, friends, family members, and co-workers added to the pile of conflicting emotions with the following comments:

- *I don't see what the big deal is—I had a hysterectomy.*
- *How can you live with that gross thing in your belly?*
- *You are soooo lucky. I would love to have a hysterectomy. I can't wait until menopause when this stupid menstrual cycle is a done deal.*
- *Think of all the time you'll get to take off from work.*
- *I made the adjustments. Why should you be any different?*
- *Are you nuts looking at other procedures? You get what you deserve if you choose anything other than a hysterectomy.*

The one comment that actually meant a great deal to me and helped me shape my decision came from a co-worker. She had undergone hysterectomy about ten years previously and was still struggling to balance her hormones. Overall, she was satisfied with her hysterectomy but admitted to me that her sex life just wasn't quite what it had been previously. The following was the sage advice from a woman who truly cared about me that I will never forget:

"Carla, if I had had another option available to me that would have allowed me to avoid a hysterectomy, I would have definitely chosen it. You can live through a hysterectomy and go on to have a good life. But that doesn't mean it's the same. It's not. You can't put anything back once it's taken out, and you don't really know how it will all turn out or how much work it will be getting your life back after the surgery. If you have another option available to you, definitely look into it. I would, if I could."

And with that, I did.

As you can see, a lot of variables contribute to the process of making "the decision." Uterine artery embolization was MY CHOICE—based on *my reasoning* and *my medical situation.* Your choice **should be just that.** *Your choice.*

Nine

Keeping a Journal

When I started out on my medical journey, I didn't really have a *journal*, so to speak. Not at all, unfortunately. If something crossed my mind that I thought was important to write down, I would grab just about any kind of paper available and start scribbling. Medical notes, phone conversations, copies of lab reports—all were stuffed in a folder in no particular order. Consequently, the journal I kept was actually a pile of odd-shaped slips of paper. Over time, the stack became unruly. I did, at least, remember to date the scraps of paper at the top of each one as I went along. But what a mess!

What I didn't understand about this mess of medical notes that was building up was that it was truly hindering my ability to see how my uterine fibroids and their symptoms were progressing. In addition, over many years it was difficult to keep track of all the tests, doctors, illnesses, and serious medical events that occurred. We moved to different states a couple of times, and new doctors would ask me questions about my medical history. Oh, brother! I would have to go home and dig for an answer. I couldn't remember it all.

The purchase of a computer along the way helped me to organize some of this information. I created a single file that I could open up and simply add to whenever I felt like it. Over time, a terrific flowchart of symptoms and events emerged. But it still didn't help me much when I was sitting in a doctor's office and wanting to take notes to refer to later.

In the end, I decided that I needed to get organized and put things in a proper sequence of events in a single binder. It was the only way that I knew I could properly track all the information that was quickly building up about my medical condition. In my case, I ended up purchasing a monthly planner with extra sheets for taking notes in the doctor's office and a three-hole sleeve pocket for each month to store those odd-shaped slips of medical papers. I didn't abandon my computer. Instead, I used it to create a table of events that could be tracked across the entire year. (*In addition, I eventually used it to transfer all my notes online and into the* **My Journal** *web pages on my website. This doesn't have to be one of your goals— but sharing this information with others online has also proved useful to me in my medical journey!*)

Information about your ongoing personal health and any problems you encounter, diagnostic tests you undergo, or procedures performed are all valuable pieces of information for your physician. In addition, keeping a running journal of all these events allows you to develop an ongoing list of questions that you can ask during the next appointment.

Before every appointment these days, I put together a short synopsis of everything I think is important that came up with my medical health since my last appointment. I create a separate list of any questions that have come up. I know. It all sounds so . . . *anal-retentive*. It probably is. But it's also a wonderful tool to assist your doctor with your care.

Obviously, no physician *requires* you to gather this information, but it sure speeds up the communication of any outstanding issues. It also opens the door to actually allow time to *talk* about those issues instead of spending so much time identifying them all while the doctor sits and takes notes.

Once upon a time, I left my doctor's office with unanswered questions that would be remembered only after I returned home. Not anymore. Keeping a journal is an invaluable tool for organization and ongoing communication with doctors.

Whether you choose to keep a journal or not is up to you. I highly recommend it, and would like to share with you a piece of my own journal that covers the year following my uterine artery embolization. While reviewing the information in my table, think about this resource and how it might be helpful to you and your doctor. Then, consider visiting your local stationery store and building your own binder to keep track of all your own personal medical information. In the end, I know you'll be glad you did.

My Journal

The following is an example of the chart I put together and followed for one year. Because I was planning to undergo uterine artery embolization, I decided to list all the symptoms I was experiencing and track them over time to determine whether or not any of them improved after the procedure. After the UAE, I discovered I needed to add a few rows for symptoms that were caused by either the UAE or medication prescribed at the same time. *To read more of* **My Journal,** *you can visit my website on the Internet.*

Prior to undergoing any procedure, and in order to track a more accurate picture of your symptoms and progress with treatments, you may choose to create your own list and track this kind of information on a monthly basis.

Symptomology	*Pre-UAE*	*6 WEEKS* *11 December 1998*	*6 MONTHS* *29 April 1999*	*1 YEAR* *2 November 1999*
Bulk of fibroid	HUGE Ultrasound report shows: uterus: 20.1 x 10 x 11.8 cm; primary Fibroid: 11.9 cm.	Still significant, but shrinkage noted by gyn. From 20–22+ weeks to 16–18 weeks in size.	Although still quite large, significantly smaller to me. Ultrasound report shows: uterus: 17 x 8.9 x 10.7 cm; primary Fibroid: 8.9 x 5.5 x 7.9 cm	Seems less. But still slightly protruding from abdomen Uterus: 17.2 x 8.1 x 7.1 Primary Fibroid: 7.8 x 7.1 x 8 Report shows relatively no change in vertical length of fibroid uteri during past 6 months but some change in width—this pretty much confirms what it feels like as well. Still big. But no longer bothersome.
Bleeding	During monthly period only. Clotting. Heavy. Just about own stock in tampon/pad market . . .	Not reduced by UAE. Bleeding continues and is now occurring "off" cycle as well as on.	First normal period at month 5 post UAE. Lasted 5 days, light flow, no clots. Month 6 the same. Cramping is, however, extensive.	Generally last about 5 days. Some clots. Cramping not bad.

Symptomology	Pre-UAE	6 WEEKS 11 December 1998	6 MONTHS 29 April 1999	1 YEAR 2 November 1999
Back pain	Excruciating. Debilitating. Living on painkillers. Narcotics and OTC drugs. Whatever I can get.	Still significant.	No longer twenty-four/ seven. Still present at excruciating levels but less frequent. Generally controlled through Motrin. "Creaking" in lower back quite common along with the feeling of knotted and pulled muscles.	Dwindled down to minor aches and pains. True back pain occurring only once every other week or so. Controlled with Motrin.
Sex	Possible. But, barely. Relieves back pain. Amazed that uterine orgasms continue even with the size of my uterus. Irregular bleeding begins post-sex in June '98.	Libido high (possibly higher then pre-UAE). Sexual "feelings" non-existent, however. No orgasms of any kind. Feels "dead." Sometimes it's "almost" and then nothing. Extremely unhappy and angry.	Libido still high. Some improvement in "feelings" and clitoral orgasms. Uterine orgasms nonexistent. "Dead weight" in the abdomen.	Libido still high. No additional improvements since 6-month mark.

Symptomology	Pre-UAE	6 WEEKS 11 December 1998	6 MONTHS 29 April 1999	1 YEAR 2 November 1999
Mental/ Emotional	Depressed to such depths that spouse never leaves me alone.	Angry. Not happy with state of bleeding, back pain, vision loss, or sex. Relieved that I've "done something" but impatient for that something to change my health and mental state.	Marked improvement. Depression fairly non-existent.	Wow. Major difference from a year ago! Can't believe how much suffering with uterine fibroids that I put myself through. Seems totally nuts looking back on it. Definite positive outlook for the future.
Migranes	Daily. Consume around 200 extra-strength Excedrine *monthly.* Frequently retreat to dark room for relief and go to bed by 7 P.M. nightly.	Gone. Not a single migraine in 6 weeks.	Still gone. Haven't purchased or taken Excedrin in 6 months.	Still gone.

Symptomology	Pre-UAE	6 WEEKS 11 December 1998	6 MONTHS 29 April 1999	1 YEAR 2 November 1999
Urinary incontinence	I scope out bathrooms everywhere I go. Bladder is definitely pressed for space.	No longer an issue.	Still no longer an issue.	Not an issue. ☺
Energy Level	Nonexistent. In bed by 7 P.M. nightly. No exercise or extra-curricular activities. Barely can make it through an evening program at my children's school.	Improved. Kind of like somebody suddenly popped a rubber band across the room—the momentum from being wound up for so long and then suddenly being released is incredible. Start going to the gym every night for a 1–2 hour workout.	More energy than everyone in my family except my 7-year-old. Repair bicycle for riding. Rollerblade. Serious swimming and upper body-building begins.	High. Unbelievably.

Symptomology	Pre-UAE	6 WEEKS 11 December 1998	6 MONTHS 29 April 1999	1 YEAR 2 November 1999
Hyperplasia/ synthetic progesterone	Began taking a synthetic progesterone 1 month pre-UAE because of hysteroscopy report showing hyperplasia without atypia.	At 6 weeks post-UAE, I've been taking synthetic progesterone for a little over 2 months. May be cause of many of my symptoms.	No longer using synthetic progesterone. Stopped at 4 months post-UAE after 5 months of prescriptive use. Recent endometrial biopsy shows proliferation of estrogen in the endrometrium—but no hyperplasia. I'm only "off" synthetic progesterone for a couple of weeks when the emotional roller coaster begins. I purchase a jar of progesterone cream and begin using it. Within days I notice the difference.	Hasn't returned.

Symptomology	Pre-UAE	6 WEEKS 11 December 1998	6 MONTHS 29 April 1999	1 YEAR 2 November 1999
Vision loss	Wear glasses. Impaired distance vision since around age 10. Myopia and astigmatism.	Some vision loss as a result of UAE or drugs or extreme pressure due to pain. Not sure which. Peripheral impacted for about 9 days but then returned to normal—night and distance vision also impacted and continues to be a problem at 6 weeks.	No improvement. Distance vision is particularly worse during performance of any kind of physical activity (bicycling, treadmill, aerobics, etc.)	Vision care not covered by insurance. Can't afford to see recommended neuro-opthalmologist. Adjusting to vision problems but still having difficulties.
Sugar Intolerance	Geez. Craved and ate sugar as frequently as possible.	Can't tolerate sweets of any kind.	Still can't tolerate sweets. No cravings or desires for food made primarily with sugar at all.	Getting better but still fairly intolerable. Definitely do not crave sweets these days.

Symptomology	Pre-UAE	6 WEEKS 11 December 1998	6 MONTHS 29 April 1999	1 YEAR 2 November 1999
Chocolate	Ate tons. Daily	Makes me want to vomit. Ugh.	Can tolerate in small quantities—like a Hershey's Kiss or two at a time—but no more. Nauseates me.	Blech.
Nausea	Nonexistent.	Daily	Only occurs with consumption of sweets.	Only occurs with consumption of sweets.
Weight	-194	-175	-152	-146
Clothing size	18++	16	10	10
Shoe size	6½	5½ For years I've been buying shoes an entire size too large because of edema. Unbelievable.	5½	5½

If this journal example seems like too much work for you to put together, there are other options available to you that will make this project a little bit easier. If you have access to the Internet, a number of medical websites now offer the ability of storing online medical records for you—for free! A really good example is My Health Record on WebMD at: **http://my.webmd.com/my_health_record**

If you don't have access to the Internet, there are a number of journal tools currently available at your local bookstore. One of the best record-keeping tools currently available is *The Savard Health Record: A Six-Step System for Managing Your Healthcare,* created by Dr. Marie Savard. This health record maintenance tracking tool comes in its own binder with preprinted forms and an excellent explanation of how to read laboratory reports.

Conclusion

These past few years I have been on the most incredible journey to finding better health. After years and years of suffering with uterine fibroids, I can honestly say that I have read nearly every book ever published on the topic, requested and read hundreds upon hundreds of reports published in the medical literature, and visited thousands of medical web pages on the Internet. After years of stumbling around in the total dark trying to figure out what to do, I finally found a solution to *my* medical dilemma. I didn't create the solution. I merely stumbled upon it: *uterine artery embolization.*

I know, with little doubt, that it was the right solution for *me.* I'm alive today, and it feels good. I am **not** promoting UAE as a solution for *you*—only *you* can figure out which path your medical journey will take you down. Perhaps it's UAE, perhaps it's myomectomy, perhaps it's even hysterectomy. What I am trying to say as simply as possible is that, after fourteen years of suffering with uterine fibroids, UAE came along at the right time and was the right solution for *me.*

It pains me terribly to look back upon my life only a short while ago to a time when I was preparing my will and writing love letters to members of my family. I was, in the manner of actions, preparing for death. How did uterine fibroids come to consume my life and take away even the most precious desires that I had for living and loving my husband and children? I don't know. They just did.

I would never wish my circumstances upon anyone, but it has been made abundantly clear to me through my work on the Internet that there are many, many women who are suffering today much as I was in 1998. Some are in even worse condition than I was. It's time, ladies—time to reach out and get the help you need to deal with your uterine fibroids. Another author might simply give you the information to read and nothing more. That's not me. There are a lot of women in this world reaching out to you with helping hands. If you are a long-term sufferer of uterine fibroids, you need to know that there are women and doctors who truly do want to help you.

The Internet

An absolutely incredible portion of my medical journey came from the outpouring of care and support that I found, of all places, on the Internet: in cyberspace.

As a technical writer for the software industry, I've known about the Internet since its birth. What I didn't know was that while I was using it as a basic research tool, other people had begun congregating in special meeting places online. Talking. Together. Sometimes all at once. Sometimes in a cyberspace auditorium of sorts. Sometimes one on one. Sometimes in *real time*. Like in a telephone call. Sometimes in email.

With the help of my teenage daughter, I learned about chat rooms, and message boards, and list groups. I began to wander in and out of all of these places online, making a lot of friends along the way who were doing the same. Looking for answers, taking a helping hand wherever it was offered, and giving a helping hand back whenever possible.

Sometime after undergoing UAE, I decided to start a new list group where women, men, and health professionals could share information on uterine fibroids. It was at that list group where a number of us came together to begin building a home site where women could come with their cup of tea and sit and read and write to one another about *their* journey. The following was placed online at the entrance of our list group to introduce people to what we are all about and to invite new members.

> ## *Group Description:*
>
> The Uterine Fibroids discussion group is for those interested in research-ing and discussing all methods of treatment for uterine fibroids. It en-courages both positive and negative feedback on all methods of treatment ranging from hysterectomy, myomectomy, uterine artery embolization (UAE), endometrial ablation, myolysis, RU-486, female reconstructive surgery (FRS), hormone replacement therapy (HRT) and any other treat-ment option that a woman may be considering or have already undergone in an effort to treat her uterine fibroids.

Over the last year, our membership has soared. Nearly every single day, a new person has subscribed to our discussion group and brought with her her own story—pieces of her own journey.

After a while, I started toying with the idea of creating a website dedi-cated to helping other women with their uterine fibroids. I learned that "homesteading" was something that went on out in cyberspace. So, I de-cided to check out the territory. In the end, I bought a little piece of air and a whole lot of bytes (computer bytes, that is) moved in, and made a home at http://www.uterinefibroids.com. This website was created specifically for women with uterine fibroids. Visitors to the site will find a HUGE collection of web links and medical information (including hot links to any bibliography item found in this book that are available for reading on the Internet!), and my very own medical journey is painstak-ingly detailed in **My Journal** online there.

Why did I do all that work developing a website? Why did I bother to write this book? Once online, I discovered hundreds upon hundreds upon *thousands* of women who were *just like me*. My mind boggles at the sheer volume of email, snail mail (you know—mail sent through the U.S. Postal Service), and telephone calls that continue to come in as a result of the uterinefibroids website. No, I'm not the only woman who has had to deal with uterine fibroids. Neither are you. Not by a long shot.

So Let's Talk

We can help ourselves move along in our medical journey and find solutions together if we only reach out and talk to one another. For too long the medical world of gynecological "female problems" has been bottled up and not discussed openly. Not even among women. Sometimes not even among best friends. Too many of us believe that we are alone in our suffering because no one talks about this health problem called uterine fibroids.

In reality, the reproductive system along with sexual function is entirely off-limits as a discussion topic—that is, unless you're having a baby or joking around with "the guys." But when was the last time you had a real conversation that included any of the following words: *uterus, ovary, cervix, fallopian tube, orgasm, clitoris, vagina, hysterectomy, myomectomy, fibroid embolization,* or even *uterine fibroids?* If you *do* happen to remember a recent conversation using any of these words (medical conversations with doctors do NOT count!), were you *whispering* at any point during the discussion? If so, why? Is there something wrong with those words? Are they bad words? Are they words we should be ashamed of? In an open conversation, why do we whisper or mumble these words? Or, more likely, not speak them at all?

It's time to realize that over one hundred fifty years of being locked up in the house with our uterine fibroids and not talking about this issue *to anyone* has gone on for far too long. The only way to make headway is to open that front door (your mouth) and start talking. Our reproductive system and our sexual functioning are part of who we are. They are a part of every man and woman on this planet. Why should you or I be ashamed or embarrassed to discuss these topics openly?

As a matter of my OWN opinion, if anyone or any group of people should be embarrassed about anything, it's the gynecological community. I know there are good doctors. But 150 years of little to no progress on determining a cause and a cure is not exactly something to write home to mother about and I will not apologize to anyone for the way I feel about this lack of progress. It's shameful.

In case you were wondering, I'm not the kind of person to whine and complain on the job without actively working on a solution. I don't have any intention of attacking the gynecological community and then turning and running. This issue is way too important to me. It demands attention and it demands solutions: better ones than hysterectomy.

Here's one element of my proposed solution: Let's talk about it. Let's get men talking about it. Let's get more and more researchers talking about it. Let's work together to make it very clear to the medical community that we want answers—not a new way to perform a hysterectomy!

Tuck whatever embarrassment or humiliation you might be feeling about the problems you are encountering with uterine fibroids into your back pocket, put on a warm overcoat, and open that door to communication. Start by truly taking the time to talk to your partner and loved ones and then move on from there.

At this point, this mom (yes, me) has three extremely well educated children who know what uterine fibroids are and know why Mommy has been so sick. In talking about my uterine fibroids with them, I discovered that *they were relieved to learn that my health and mental well-being weren't based on something they did.* If you have children and you have never talked to them about your health before, I urge you to do so. Sharing lots of medical detail isn't really important. Simply discussing your health with them *is* important. You might be surprised at how much they love you and want you to be well. You might also be surprised at how worried they are about you. Talk to them. Maybe one of your children will be part of the next generation of doctors and researchers who will find a solution to this problem. Love is a strong motivator.

We can open that door to communication if we really want to. We can even find solutions *together,* if we only reach out and talk to one another.

The Men Survey

On many women's list groups and across a wide variety of message boards, women frequently wonder about men and the choices they are presented with from the medical community versus the choices they themselves, as women, have been presented with from their doctors. Comments like the following one, written by a woman several years after her hysterectomy, are extremely common to read from time to time on message boards:

"I believe the uterus continues to function for life, well after childbearing years and menopause. Its usefulness doesn't end just because you don't want

*any more children. If a man has to have his prostate (or any sexual organ) re-moved, the question of having a child is probably the LAST question asked—if it's asked at all. The first concern is sexual function. Why is a man's sexual function so much more important than a woman's? This double standard needs to come to an end. Doctors have told me that removing a woman's uterus has no impact on sex. But that has not been **my** experience."*

This message, along with many others, made me wonder about men's versus women's choices too. Indeed, the following statement made by Dr. Scott Goodwin in *Imaging News* (April 1998) also caught my interest:

"I don't think that much attention's being paid to the psychological impact that hysterectomy can have ... Sometimes I wonder how much attention would be garnered if most of the urologists in this country were women and they were performing 600,000 orchiectomies a year."

This type of observational commentary made by women and physicians alike made me wonder why more men weren't involved in the health and well-being of their female partners. Certainly the reproductive and sexual health of women has an impact on the relationship with their male partners, doesn't it? So why do men just sit back and not get involved with the decisions that their female counterparts are making? Or, worse yet, why do some men PUSH women into having procedures—particularly hysterectomy? (Yes. It happens.) Would the hysterectomy and oophorectomy statistics change at all if more men were involved in the treatment choices women make about their uterine fibroids?

In trying to find an answer to some of these questions, I began re-searching the prostate and, much to my surprise, discovered that about 375,000 men enter the hospital each year for an enlarged prostate gland. In addition, doctors seem to know about as much about an enlarged prostate gland as they do about a fibroid uterus.

It shouldn't have surprised me, but the following fact certainly did: In 10 percent of all cases of enlarged prostate glands, the tissue removed is found to have some cancer cells. Additional surgery, however, is NOT done or even suggested to men as a method of preventing the recurrence of those cancer cells. (It's a slow-growing cancer supposedly making pre-ventive surgery unnecessary.) Compare that to the roughly 360,000 women who have their ovaries removed for the *prevention* of ovarian cancer *every year*—when the liftime risk of cancer was only 1.8 percent.

The differences in how the medical community treats men and women don't end there. What about the issue of sexual function? How is men's sexual function treated differently than women's? When cancer is present in the prostate glands of men, sometimes (no, not always) the testes are removed. This is called *orchiectomy*. If both testes are removed, this is called *bilateral orchiectomy* or *castration*. Sound familiar? It should. It is the surgical and hormonal equivalent of bilateral oophorectomy in women—the removal of both ovaries.

The big difference is that it is awfully hard to find the word *castration* in women's health books and even harder yet to get that word out of a doctor's mouth. But I found it in nearly every medical reference to orchiectomy that I came across right along with the recommendation for testosterone hormone replacement therapy. On top of that, there were often entries such as this one found in the Healtheon Corporation's online medical dictionary:

> "He will need help in dealing with problems related to his masculinity, self-concept, and sexual activity. He should be given time to think about and discuss the effects of his surgery."

That quote came out of a medical *dictionary*.

In checking the very same medical dictionary for the word *oophorectomy*, a reference to the term *castration* was nowhere to be seen. In addition, there was no recommendation for hormone replacement therapy, and there was no patient care advice (as with the statement above for orchiectomy) at all.

Yes, the medical community measures and treats men differently than it does women. The above example can be found over and over again in medical documentation. It is not a singular anomaly. One woman wrote to me to say that she was so shocked at her doctor's recommendation for the removal of her ovaries with an upcoming hysterectomy that she blurted out, *"But, Doc—isn't that castration?"* His answer? A brusque *"No. It's not."* She pushed him on this issue and asked about the hormones that the ovaries produce and wondered about her sexual drive. He ended the meeting by getting up and walking out and then sending her a certified letter indicating he no longer wished to be her physician.

Consider the same scenario with a man talking to his doctor about orchiectomy. Who do you think would get up and leave the room, never to return?

It was that thought that drove me to develop the **Men Survey.** A number of women batted it around a bit on the uterinefibroids list group, and it was ultimately turned into a survey that could be emailed to men. (It's also available online at the www.uterinefibroids.com website.) It's purpose was/is to both solicit information from men on this subject AND to enlighten and inform them about the similar health choices that women are presented with in regard to their reproductive and sexual organs. (A copy of the **Men Survey** can be found on page 231.)

There were five basic questions asked of men that all dealt with a doctor's recommendation for orchiectomy because of the *potential* for cancer. All of the questions ended with "Now what do you do or say?"

The **Men Survey** was initially emailed to over two thousand people. Women, men, and medical professionals received this survey. From there, it was forwarded countless times. One woman liked it so much she declared, *"I sent a copy to each of my ex-husbands! None of them ever 'got it'—perhaps they will now."*

The response was tremendous. Men sent me all kinds of personal stories and elaborate scenarios that told me they *could* relate to this situation. They also cussed, gave statistics, and unequivocally and unanimously responded with "No. No. No. No. No." Five questions with five pretty clear answers. *"No, you may **NOT** remove my testicles!"* Not a single man responded otherwise or even waffled a bit on this issue. Other answers included the following:

- Why do I need *this* procedure? Are there any alternative treatments?
- I have a good chance of dying in an automobile accident, too. Should I quit driving?
- Would I be able to have a normal sex life?
- I really need to think about it. I take your input very seriously and I understand the seriousness of the diagnosis. But this is a serious decision and I don't make major decisions hastily.
- Yes, I do want to be around for my children. This is no reason for such a drastic surgery is it?
- Why should I have a major (elective) surgery for something that is a *risk* but not inevitable? No, I don't think so.

In addition to responding to the questions asked, heartfelt email that responded directly to the **Footnote** information at the bottom of the survey was also received. It told me that men read the information. It told me that men cared. It told me that men are willing to be educated on this issue if we only choose to discuss it with them. Here's a typical response that was received:

"I believe that this is a serious issue that we face and that women all over need to be aware there are other options. Also I think in situations like this a "patient advocate" would be a very wise thing for the patient to check into simply because the psychological trauma presented to a person in this circumstance would be overwhelming. (Whether they are male or female.) Too many patients hold their doctors next to God himself. They *are* fallible. They are human."

As I stated previously, the **Men Survey** was also sent to women: a thousand or so. Many of the responses received were from women who had undergone hysterectomy with bilateral salpingo-oophorectomy. Most women were supportive of this educational effort directed at men. Nonetheless, there were some who were angry with me for making light of such a serious topic as *female castration*. Because of their own struggles and poor outcome from oophorectomy, they were angry and could not see their way clear to any educational value of this survey for men. Others were sad. Some were reflective. Too many were like this one:

"In answer to why do so many women agree to this surgery? I don't know about the other women who will have it done this year, but I agreed after two years of my doctor telling me it was no big deal and I was a big baby to not give in and have this wonderful surgery that would make me 'feel like a million bucks' . . . in short, the man lied . . . even when I asked questions, he lied . . . "

Good Doctors—Are There Any?

If you've read all the way through this book, you may have come to believe that I am not particularly fond of gynecologists.

In the course of treating my fibroids, I've had more than my fair share of gynecologists who were not interested in my long-term health and well-being and who certainly were not interested in carrying on any kind of conversation with me. Based on some of the recommendations I received for hysterectomy, it was pretty clear to me that the doctor's pocketbook was held in much higher esteem than my body. Even so, there *are* good doctors out there.

It took me awhile to figure out that I just wasn't doing my homework in trying to locate a good doctor. Finding a good doctor is about a lot more than opening an HMO book or the yellow pages and calling the first number your index finder lands on. I bet you know this technique. It goes something like this: You open the book, close your eyes, and point downward until your finger touches the page. *Violà!* New doctor. I knew it! You have used that technique. You can't lie to me. I've been there and done that.

But you know what? With every bad doctor I encountered, I kept pushing. Pulling. Asking questions. Looking for answers. Talking to other women who DID seem to have good doctors. Then I started asking *doctors* the best question out there: How does someone know whether or not a doctor is a "good" doctor? Would you like to know something? Doctors do know the answer to this question. Even bad doctors usually know the answer to this question! But you have to ask first. Much of the information in chapter 8, *Making a Decision,* was based on information that I picked up from *doctors.*

So today I'm happy to say that I'm surrounded by good doctors. Some of the best. Are they supergods of the medical world? Nope. They're human. They make mistakes just as I do. The difference is, they're willing to talk about it. *They're willing to be human.* They're even willing to actually have a conversation *with* me—not *at* me—about my health. I like that. I find *trust* in that. Wouldn't you?

Best of all, they acknowledge the path I've journeyed on and they empathize with me. They do NOT take offense when painful memories surface and cause me to verbally slam gynecology or gynecologists as a whole. I'll admit they physically cringe a bit sometimes, but they do not take offense and they do give me room to simply vent and get it out.

Yes, Virginia. There is a Santa Claus. Good doctors are everywhere. Unfortunately, so are the bad ones. I can't say it often enough . . . DO YOUR HOMEWORK!

*Wishing you all the best on **your** journey,*

Carla

Appendices

National Uterine Fibroids Foundation

On March 22, 2000, the National Uterine Fibroids Foundation (NUFF) was borne. This organization is dedicated to the education, care, and treatment of women who have uterine fibroids or related conditions of the reproductive system. In founding this nonprofit organization, it is my hope that we can truly build a support system for women at the same time that we are pushing forth the research that would unlock the answers to this disease. *"I've simply had 'nuff now I'd like some research!"*

The purpose and long-term goals of this organization are:

➤ To **provide information to the public** about the diagnosis of, and treatment options for, uterine fibroids and related conditions affecting women's reproductive systems, and the right to receive, and the nature of, informed consent from medical providers for the treatment of uterine fibroids and related medical conditions affecting women's reproductive systems;

➤ To **advocate for the rights** of all women to maintain independent choice in the matter of deciding upon treatment options for uterine fibroids and related medical conditions affecting women's reproductive systems;

➤ To **facilitate research studies conducted on the cause of, treatment options for, and patient outcomes associated with treat-**

ment of uterine fibroids and related medical conditions, so as to increase the body of scientific knowledge and access thereto by, among other things, funding research studies; creating, maintaining, and making publicly available a database of research materials and information on current or ongoing research studies; and creating, maintaining, and making publicly available databases of medical providers, researchers and patients, so as to facilitate contact between the scientific and medical community and patients, as well as to provide a forum for members of the scientific and medical community to meet one another and to share information in an effort to undertake specialty-specific and interdisciplinary research studies;

➤ To **promote alternatives to hysterectomy** in an effort to thereby reduce the number of unnecessary hysterectomies performed on women with gynecological problems each year in the United States;

➤ To **provide support** to internet-developed women's health groups that provide services to women recovering from treatment choices that resulted in a negative outcome and/or reduced Quality of Life related to uterine fibroids and/or other conditions of their reproductive systems.

In order to fulfill these goals, the National Uterine Fibroids Foundation will need YOUR help. For more information, please contact NUFF at:

National Uterine Fibroids Foundation
1132 Lucero Street
Camarillo, CA 93010
1-877-553-NUFF
(805) 482-2698
Email address: info@NUFF.org
website: http://www.NUFF.org

Treating the Symptoms of Uterine Fibroids

The following table is offered as a quick synopsis of all treatment options for the symptoms of uterine fibroids and does not, necessarily, represent all benefits and risks for any one treatment option. Please read chapter 5 for a more complete discussion of each option presented below.

Symptom	Treatment Options	Benefits	Risks
Abnormal bleeding (*resulting in anemia, fatigue, etc.*)	Ignore it.	Avoids medical intervention of all kinds.	Fatigue Anemia Could become life threatening. May signal a precancerous condition.
	Vitex (chaste berry)	May reduce bleeding.	May cause stomachaches, skin rash, and itching. Slow-acting herb that may take 3–6 months to work. May not help bleeding.
	False unicorn	May reduce bleeding.	Usually taken with Vitex and no proof exists that this medicine based in Native American tradition works. May not help bleeding.

Symptom	Treatment Options	Benefits	Risks
	Dilation and curettage (D&C)	Provides tissue for cancer analysis. May temporarily control bleeding.	May not help bleeding.
	Nonsteroidal anti-inflammatory drugs (NSAIDs), progestins, GnRH agonists	May control bleeding.	Take at least a month to work.
	Endometrial ablation	Controls bleeding 70 to 90 percent of time.	Long-term side effects not known.
Chronic pelvic pain or pressure	Nonsteroidal anti-inflammatory drugs (NSAIDs)	May control pain.	NSAIDs can irritate stomach.
	Oral contraceptives	May control pain.	May cause fluid retention and weight gain.

Symptom	Treatment Options	Benefits	Risks
	Exercise	May strengthen muscles supporting uterus and fibroids. Increases endorphins in system and may contribute to overall sense of well-being.	May not help.
	Psychological counseling	Offers insight into pain and coping techniques.	May not help.
Constipation	Laxatives	May help relieve bulk and pressure of constipation.	Not a long-term solution as physical dependency may occur.
	Increase fiber intake	May help relieve bulk. Healthy long-term option.	May take time to relieve symptom.

Treatment Options for Uterine Fibroid Tumors

The following table is offered as a quick synopsis of all treatment options and does not, necessarily, represent all benefits and risks for any one treatment option. Please read chapter 6 for a more complete discussion of each option presented below.

Treatment	Location	Size	Benefits	Risks
Gonadotropin-releasing hormone (*GnRH*) *agonists* (*Nafarelin, Leuprolide—Lupron*)	Any	Any	Decreases bleeding. Shrinks fibroids.	May cause symptoms of early menopause (hot flashes, vaginal dryness, mood swings). Can be severe. Fibroids return once treatment is discontinued—but long-term use is NOT recommended due to a myriad of nondesirable side effects including a potentially severe bone marrow loss leading to osteoporosis. Not approved by the FDA for anything other than improving preoperative bleeding. Costly.

Treatment	Location	Size	Benefits	Risks
Hysteroscopic Myomectomy (*surgical removal of fibroid tumors*)—*vaginal entrance*	Submucosal	Varies	Surgical removal of fibroids. Controls bleeding and pressure symptoms. Can be done on an outpatient basis. Minimal recovery time.	Tumors recur in about 30 percent of women within five years, requiring additional treatment 10 percent of the time.
Laparoscopic Myomectomy (*surgical removal of fibroid tumors*)—*small puncture entrances through navel and abdomen*	Subserosal Pedunculated	Varies	Surgical removal of fibroids. Controls bleeding and pressure symptoms. Can be done on an outpatient basis. Minimal recovery time	Tumors recur in about 30 percent of women within five years, requiring additional treatment 10 percent of the time.

Treatment	Location	Size	Benefits	Risks
Laparotomy-Abdominal Myomectomy *(surgical removal of fibroid tumors)— abdominal incision*	Intramural Subserosal Pedunculated	Any	Surgical removal of fibroids. Controls bleeding and pressure symptoms.	Major surgery Tumors recur in about 30 percent of women within five years, requiring additional treatment 10 percent of the time. requiring hysterectomy. Complications during procedure Uncontrollable leakage of urine Injury to bladder Injury to ureter Injury to the bowel and/or intestinal obstruction Sterility Pulmonary embolism
Uterine Artery Embolization (UAE) (Not recommended when endometriosis is present.)	Any	Any	Noninvasive, nonsurgical procedure	Complete symptom resolution may take six months to a year.

Treatment	Location	Size	Benefits	Risks
			Short recovery time Controls bleeding and pressure symptoms. Current studies show **no** signs of tumor recurrence.	Menopause (This procedure is NOT recommended for women desiring a future pregnancy.) Infection resulting in hysterectomy Bleeding not resolved in 2 to 4 percent of all cases. Internal uterine/cervical sexual or-gasms *may* be impacted. May not be covered by insurance.
Myolysis (*not recommended when endometriosis or adenomyosis is present*)	Subserosal. Pedunculated	No larger than 10 cm and no more than 4–5 fibroids	Controls bleeding and pressure symptoms.	May require pretreatment with a GnRH. Infection resulting in hysterectomy

Treatment	Location	Size	Benefits	Risks
Cryomyolysis (*Not recommended when endometriosis or adenomyosis is present.*)	Subserosal Pedunculated	No larger than 10 cm and no more than 4–5 fibroids	Controls bleeding and pressure symptoms.	May require pretreatment with a GnRH. Infection resulting in hysterectomy.
Subtotal Hysterectomy (*Uterus only removed through the abdomen.*)	Any	Any	Curative. Removal of all fibroids along with the uterus Internal uterine/cervical-related sexual orgasms may *not* be impacted—research is inconclusive on this.	Major surgery Loss of uterine-contractions-related sexual orgasms Injury to bladder Injury to ureters Injury to the bowel and/or intestinal obstruction Ovarian failure occurs 20 percent of the time when ovaries are retained (only 40 percent of all women currently retain their ovaries with hysterectomy).

Treatment	Location	Size	Benefits	Risks
Total Hysterectomy (*Uterus and cervix removed abdominally or vaginally.*)	Any	For vaginal removal, uterus/fibroids must be small enough to fit through vaginal opening.	Curative. Removal of all fibroids along with the uterus	Major surgery Uncontrollable leakage of urine Injury to bladder Injury to ureters Injury to the bowel and/or intestinal obstruction Formation of fistula between vagina and rectum Ovarian failure Painful intercourse Loss of uterine-contractions-related sexual orgasms
Radical Hysterectomy (*Reserved for serious disease such as cancer. Uterus, cervix, fallopian tubes, ovaries, and pelvic lymph nodes removed through the abdomen.*)	Any	Any	Curative for fibroids. May be curative for cancer.	Major surgery Damage to other organs—such as the bladder—resulting in need for additional reparative surgery Surgical menopause May not be curative for cancer Loss of uterine-related sexual orgasms

Related Health Issues

The following table is offered as a quick synopsis of the related health issues presented in Chapter 7 and does not, necessarily, represent all benefits and risks of treatment for any one health issue. Please read Chapter 7 for a more complete discussion of each issue presented here.

Symptom	Treatment Options	Benefits	Risks
Adenomyosis	Hysterectomy	Curative	Complications of hysterectomy
	Uterine artery embolization	May be curative.	May not help. Research still in progress.
Cancer (endometrial cancer, cervical cancer, leiomyosarcoma, ovarian cancer)	Total hysterectomy Radical hysterectomy	May be curative.	Complications of hysterectomy May not "cure" cancer. Surgical menopause
Dysplasia (precancerous lesions of cervix)	Cone biopsy Loop electrosurgical excision procedure (LEEP) Laser therapy Cryosurgery	Provides tissue for cancer analysis. All involve minimal pain	Cone biopsy requires general anesthesia.

Symptom	Treatment Options	Benefits	Risks
Endometriosis	Oral contraceptives	May slow growth of endometriosis.	Depending on the contraceptive, may cause any number of side effects including breast tenderness and weight gain.
	GnRH agonists	May slow growth of endometriosis.	GnRH agonists may cause symptoms of early menopause. May require some form of "addback" hormonal therapy to counter long-term impact of osteoporosis. Costly May not help.
	Danazol	May slow growth of endometriosis.	Danazol may cause excess facial hair, fluid retention, and other side effects. Costly May not help.

Symptom	Treatment Options	Benefits	Risks
Hyperplasia (*precancerous condition of the endometrial lining*)	Hysteroscopy or endometrial biopsy	Involves little pain. Provides tissue for cancer analysis.	Doesn't resolve hyperplasia.
	Dilation and curettage (D&C)	Provides tissue for cancer analysis. May resolve hyperplasia.	Hyperplasia may return by the next menstrual cycle. Perforation of uterus possible.
	Progestins	Regress hyperplasia 75 percent of the time. May control related bleeding.	May cause fluid retention and weight gain or any number of other side effects.

Symptom	Treatment Options	Benefits	Risks
Ovarian Cysts *(Cysts that show signs of being cancerous should always be removed through abdominal surgery.)*	Ignore them.	May go away on their own.	May get worse.
	Oral contraceptives	No proven benefit once cysts are formed. Can prevent new ovarian cysts from forming.	Depending on the contracepive, may cause any number of side effects including breast tenderness and weight gain.
	Remove cysts via laparoscopy.	Curative	May be necessary to remove the entire ovary.
Prolapse *("dropped uterus")*	Pelvic floor exercises	Strengthen muscles that support uterus and control urine.	May not help.
	Pessary (device worn in vagina)	Helps support uterus.	May dislodge or cause irritation. Not a long-term solution.
	Uro-gynecological surgery	Sling mesh used in surgery may help to better support uterus.	May not work. May not be a long-term solution.

Symptom	Treatment Options	Benefits	Risks
Sexual Dysfunction	Psychological counseling	Offers insight into dysfunction and coping techniques.	May not help true physiologically related sexual dysfunction.
	Viagra (Sildenafil Citrate)	May enhance blood flow/oxygen to pelvic region and increased sensitivity or intensity of orgasm.	Large clinical trials with women have not been completed that prove efficacy. Not FDA approved for use in female sexual dysfunction.
	Methyl Testosterone	May help with desire, dyspareunia, or lack of vaginal lubrication.	May cause masculine side effects, liver tumors, and other as yet unknown side effects.
	Estrogen	May improve clitoral sensitivity, increase libido and lubrication, and decrease burning and pain during intercourse.	May cause vaginal bleeding, pain in the calves or chest, severe headache, dizziness, changes in vision, breast lumps, jaundice, or mental depression.

Symptom	Treatment Options	Benefits	Risks
	Ginkgo biloba	May help to treat sexual dysfunction induced by antidepressants.	Clinical studies incomplete.
	Apomorphine, Yohimbine, L-arginine, Phentolamine (Vasomax)	May help with arousal, lubrication, and increased sensitivity or intensity of orgasm.	Clinical studies incomplete. Not approved for use in women yet. Unknown side effects of any one of these drugs may include: nasal congestion, insomnia, indigestion, increased blood pressure, etc. High number of "unknowns" as applied to women

United States Medical Boards

State	Link	Phone
Alabama	Alabama State Board of Medical Examiners 848 Washington Ave. Montgomery, AL 36104 http://www.albme.org/	334.242.4116 334.242.4155 (fax)
Alaska	Alaska State Medical Board 333 Willoughby Ave., 9th Floor Juneau, AK 99801 P.O. Box 110806 Juneau, AK 99811 http://www.dced.state.ak.us/occ/pmed.htm	907.269.8163 907.465.2541 907.465.2974 (fax)
Arizona	Arizona Board of Medical Examiners 9545 E. Doubletree Ranch Road Scottsdale, AZ 85258 http://www.docboard.org/az/df/azsearch.htm/	480.551.2700 Phoenix 877.255.2212 (toll free within AZ)

State	Link	Phone
Arkansas	Arkansas State Medical Board 2100 Riverfront Dr., Suite 200 Little Rock, AR 72202 http://www.armedicalboard.org/	501.296.1802 501.296.1805 (fax)
California	Medical Board of California 1426 Howe Ave., Suite 54 Sacramento, CA 95825 http://www.medbd.ca.gov/	916.263.2382 916.263.2487 (fax)
Colorado	Colorado State Board of Medical Examiners 1560 Broadway, Suite 1300 Denver, CO 80202-5140 http://www.dora.state.co.us/medical/	303.894.7690 303.894.7692 (fax)
Connecticut	Connecticut Department of Public Health/ Physician Licensure Department Physician Licensure	860.509.7603 860.509.8457 (fax)

State	Link	Phone
	410 Capitol Ave. Initial MS#12APP Hartford, CT 06134-0308 http://www.state.ct.us/dph/	
Delaware	Delaware Board of Medical Practice Suite 203 P.O. Box 1401 Dover, DE 19904 http://www.state.de.us/license/bomp.htm	302.739.4522 302.739.2711 (fax)
District of Columbia	District of Columbia Board of Medicine 825 N. Capital St. NE Washington, DC 20002 http://www.dchealth.com/lra/welcome.htm	202.442.9200 202.442.9431 (fax)
Florida	Florida Department of Health 4042 Bald Cypress Way Tallahassee, FL 32337 http://www.doh.state.fl.us/	850.488.0595 850.922.3040 (fax)

State	Link	Phone
Georgia	Georgia Composite State Board of Medical Examiners 166 Pryor St., SW Atlanta, GA 30303-3465 http://www.sos.state.ga.us/ebd-medical/	404.656.3913 404.656.9723 (fax)
Hawaii	Hawaii Board of Medical Examiners 1010 Richard St. Honolulu, HI 96801 P.O. Box 96813 Honolulu, HI 96813 http://www.state.hi.us/dcca/pvl/areas_medical.htm/	808.586.3000
Idaho	Idaho State Board of Medicine 280 N. 8th St., Suite 202 State House Mall Boise, ID 83720-0058 http://www.idacare.org/	208.334.2822 208.334.2801 (fax)

State	Link	Phone
Illinois	Illinois Department of Professional Regulation 320 W. Washington St., 3rd Floor Springfield, IL 62786 http://www.dpr.state.il.us/	217.785.0800 217.782.7645 (fax)
Indiana	Indiana Health Professions Bureau 402 W. Washington St., Room 41 Indianapolis, IN 46204 http://www.state.in.us/hpb/	317.232.2960 317.233.4236 (fax)
Iowa	Iowa Board of Medical Examiners 400 SW 8th St., Suite C Des Moines, IA 50309 http://www.docboard.org/ia/ia_home.htm	515.281.5171 515.242.5908 (fax)

State	Link	Phone
Kansas	Kansas State Board of Healing Arts 235 S. Topeka Blvd. Topeka, KS 66603-3068 http://www.ksbha.org	785.296.7413 785.296.0852 (fax)
Kentucky	Kentucky Board of Medical Licensure Hurstbourne Office Park 310 Whittington Pkwy, Suite 1-B Louisville, KY 40222 http://www.state.ky.us/agencies/kbml	502.429.8046 502.429.9923 (fax)
Louisiana	Louisiana State Board of Medical Examiners 630 Camp St. New Orleans, LA 70130 P.O. Box 30250 New Orleans, LA 70190-0250 http://www.lsbme.org/	504.568.6820 504.599-0503 (fax)

State	Link	Phone
Maine	Maine Board of Licensure in Medicine 137 State House Station Augusta, ME 04333 http://www.docboard.org/me/me_home.htm	207.287.3601
Maryland	Maryland Board of Physician Quality Assurance 4210 Patterson Ave. P.O. Box 2571 Baltimore, MD 21215-0002 http://www.docboard.org/md/default.htm	410.764.4777 800.492.6836 410.352.2252 (fax)
Massachusetts	Massachusetts Board of Registration in Medicine 10 West St. Boston, MA 02111 http://www.massmedboard.org/	617.727.3086

State	Link	Phone
Michigan	Michigan Board of Medicine 611 W. Ottawa, First Floor Lansing, MI 48933 P.O. Box 30670 Lansing, MI 48909 http://www.cis.state.mi.us/bhser/home.htm	517.335.0918 517.373.2179 (fax)
Minnesota	Minnesota Board of Medical Practice 2829 University Ave., SE, Suite 400 Minneapolis, MN 55414-3246 http://www.bmp.state.mn.us/	612.617.2130 612.617.2166 (fax)
Mississippi	Mississippi State Board of Medical Licensure 1867 Crane Ridge Dr., Suite 200-B Jackson, MS 39216 http://www.msbml.state.ms.us/	601.987.3079 601.987.4159 (fax)

State	Link	Phone
Missouri	Missouri State Board of Registration for the Healing Arts 3605 Missouri Blvd. Jefferson City, MO 65109 P.O. Box 4 Jefferson City, MO 65102 http://www.ecodev.state.mo.us/pr/healarts/	573.751.0098 573.571.3166 (fax)
Montana	Montana Board of Medical Examiners 301 South Park, 4th floor Helena, MT 59620-0513 P.O. Box 200513 Helena, MT 59620-0513 http://www.com.state.mt.us/license/pol/pol_boards/med_board/board_page.htm	406.444.4284 406.444.1667 (fax)

State	Link	Phone
Nebraska	Nebraska Department of Health 301 Centennial Mall South P. O. Box 95007 Lincoln, NE 68509-4986 http://www.hhs.state.ne.us/reg/regindex.htm	402.471.2115 402.471.3577 (fax)
Nevada	Nevada State Board of Medical Examiners 1105 Terminal Way, Suite 301 Reno, NV 89502 P.O. Box 7238 Reno, NV 89510 http://www.state.nv.us/medical/	702.688.2559 702.688.2321 (fax)
New Hampshire	New Hampshire Board of Medicine 2 Industrial Park Dr., Suite 8 Concord, NH 03301-8520 http://www.state.nh.us/medicine	603.271.1203 603.271.6702 (fax)
New Jersey	New Jersey State Board of Medical Examiners 140 E. Front St., 2nd Floor Trenton, NJ 08608 http://www.state.nj.us/lps/ca/medical.htm	609.826.7100 609.984.3930 (fax)

State	Link	Phone
New Mexico	New Mexico State Board of Medical Examiners 2nd Floor, Lamy Bldg. 491 Old Santa Fe Trail Santa Fe, NM 87501 http://www.healthlinknm.org/	505.827.5022 505.827.7377 (fax)
New York	New York State Board of Medicine Cultural Education Center, #3023 Albany, NY 12230 http://www.health.state.ny.us/nysdoh/opmc/main.htm	518.474.3841 518.486.4846 (fax)
North Carolina	North Carolina Board of Medical Examiners 1201 Front St., Suite 100 P.O. Box 20007 Raleigh, NC 27609 http://www.docboard.org/nc/	919.326.1100 800.253.9653 (toll free within NC) 919.326.1131 (fax)

State	Link	Phone
North Dakota	North Dakota State Board of Medical Examiners City Center Plaza 418 E. Broadway Ave., Suite 12 Bismark, ND 58501 (no website)	701.328.6500 701.328.6505 (fax)
Ohio	State Medical Board of Ohio 77 S. High St., 17th Floor Columbus, OH 43266-0315 http://www.state.oh.us/med/	614.466.3934 614.728.5946 (fax)
Oklahoma	Oklahoma State Board of Medical Licensure and Supervision 5104 N. Francis, Suite C Oklahoma City, OK 73118-6020 http://www.osbmls.state.ok.us/	405.848.6841 405.848.8240 (fax) 800.381.4519 (toll-free within OK)

State	Link	Phone
Oregon	Oregon Board of Medical Examiners 1500 SW 1st Ave., Suite 620 Portland, OR 97201 http://www.bme.state.or.us/	503.229.5770 877.254.6263 (toll free within OR) 503.229.6543 (fax)
Pennsylvania	Pennsylvania State Board of Medicine 124 Pine St. Harrisburg, PA 17101 http://www.dos.state.pa.us/bpoa/disciplinaryactions.html	717.787.8503 717.787.7769 (fax)
Rhode Island	Rhode Island Board of Medical Licensure and Discipline Cannon Bldg., Room 205 3 Capitol Hill Providence, RI 02908-5097 http://www.docboard.org/ri/main.htm	401.222.3855 401.222.2158 (fax)

State	Link	Phone
South Carolina	South Carolina Board of Medical Examiners 110 Centerview Dr., Suite 202 P.O. Box 11289 Columbia, SC 29211-1289 http://www.llr.state.sc.us./POL/Medical	803.896.4500 803.896.4515 (fax)
South Dakota	South Dakota State Board of Medical and Osteopathic Examiners 1323 S. Minnesota Ave. Sioux Falls, SC 57105 http://www.state.sd.us/dcr/medical/med-hom.htm	605.334.8343 605.336.0270 (fax)
Tennessee	Tennessee Board of Medical Examiners 1st Floor Cordell Hull Bldg. 425 5th Ave. North Nashville, TN 37247-1010 http://www.state.tn.us/health	615.741.3111 615.741.2491 (fax)

State	Link	Phone
Texas	Texas State Board of Medical Examiners 333 Guadeloupe, Tower 3, Suite 610 P.O. Box 2018 Austin, TX 78701 http://www.tsbme.state.tx.us/	800.248.4062 512.463.9416 (fax)
Utah	Utah Department of Commerce/ Division of Occupational and Professional Licensing Heber Wells Bldg., 4th Floor 160 E. 300 South P.O. Box 146741 Salt Lake City, UT 84114-6741 http://www.commerce.state.ut.us/dopl/ current/1205.htm	801.530.6628 801.530.6511 (fax)
Vermont	Vermont Board of Medical Practice 109 State St. Montpelier, VT 05609-1106 http://www.docboard.org/vt/vermont.htm	802.828.2673 802.828.5450 (fax)

State	Link	Phone
Virginia	Virginia Board of Medicine 6606 W. Broad St., 4th Floor Richmond, VA 23230-1717 http://www.dhp.state.va.us/	804.662.7636 804.662.9443 (fax)
Washington	Washington Medical Quality Assurance Commission P.O. Box 47866 1300 Quince Street SE Olympia, WA 98504-7866 http://www.doh.wa.gov/hsqa/hpqad/MQAC/default.htm	360.236.4800 360.586.4573 (fax)
West Virginia	West Virginia Board of Medicine 101 Dee Dr. Charleston, WV 25311 http://www.wvdhhr.org/wvbom/	304.558.2921 304.558.2084 (fax)

State	Link	Phone
Wisconsin	Wisconsin Medical Examining Board Dept. of Regulation and Licensing 1400 E. Washington Ave., Room 178 P.O. Box 8935 Madison, WI 53708-8935 http://badger.state.wi.us/agencies/drl/	608.266.1188 608.261.7083 (fax)
Wyoming	Wyoming Board of Medicine 211 W. 19th St. Cheyenne, WY 82002 http://soswy.state.wy.us/director/ag-bd/medicine.htm	307.778.7053 800.438.5784 (toll free) 307.778.2069 (fax)

Sample Informed Consent

TOTAL ABDOMINAL HYSTERECTOMY *

I, _____, allow Dr. _____ to perform upon me an operation known as total abdominal hysterectomy. I further understand that s/he will be assisted in performing this operation by _____, but that the major part of the operation will be performed by Dr. _____. I also understand and agree that I (initial one of the following):

_____ will

_____ will not

be used as a teaching example to train resident physicians or the medical staff. I have been informed that Dr. _____ has performed _____ (number) total abdominal hysterectomies during the last 12 months and that the mortality rate was _____, the infection rate was _____ and the complication rate was _____.

INCISION. I have been informed that a total abdominal hysterectomy is a major operation. There will be a long cut through the skin of my abdominal wall that will go through the muscles and down the inside of my abdomen. A total abdominal hysterectomy consists of the removal of the entire uterus including the main pear-shaped muscle portion of the uterus *and* the cervix.

BLOOD TRANSFUSION. As with any major surgery bleeding can occur and blood transfusions may be necessary.

INFECTION. Infection can occur. Although an infection may be superficial – just beneath the skin, it can cause a severe infection of the muscles and major infection in the pelvic portion of my abdomen. If the infection spreads, it can cause death.

URETERS. Because the ureters (by which urine passes from the kidneys to the bladder) are in such close proximity to the uterus, they may be injured during this procedure. When there is extensive disease in the pelvic area such an injury may be more common. Damage to the ureters can cause persistent leakage of urine into the vagina or into the abdomen and even damage a kidney with the possibility of infection and the necessity of its removal. Injury to the ureters may also damage both kidneys, which can cause death due to kidney failure.

BLADDER. When performing a total abdominal hysterectomy the bladder must be pushed off and cut from the lower end of the womb and the bladder may be injured. If the bladder is injured, a persistent urinary leakage may occur through the vagina or through the abdominal wall. To repair this condition additional surgery may be required.

VAGINA. Because the cervix must be removed from the vagina there may be some shortening of the vagina and chronic discomfort in the vaginal region. There may be persistent heavy discharge for a few weeks. I understand that intercourse may not be permitted for at least six to eight weeks following the operation and then only when my surgeon informs me that healing has been completed.

BLOOD CLOTS. After any operation, blood clots may occur in the leg veins. These clots may cause severe damage to my legs, resulting in subsequent varicose veins and ulcerations around the ankles. Pieces of these clots may break off and travel through my heart into the lung and cause chest pain and possibly death. After surgery the doctor will use elastic stockings on my legs and encourage me to get out of bed as soon as possible. S/he will advise me to exercise my legs in bed to diminish clot formation. Blood clots may also travel to my brain.

FERTILITY. I understand that this operation will render me sterile and unable ever to conceive children. I have also been informed that I may experience sexual arousal disorder, orgasmic disorder, or sexual pain (dyspareunia) as the result of this procedure.

OVARIES. If, during the surgical procedure, my doctor encounters a disease of the ovaries, I understand and agree that one or both ovaries (initial one of the following):

_____ may

_____ may not

Total Abdominal Hysterectomy Consent Form   Page 1 of 2

*Prepared for readers' general information. Consult an attorney licensed in your state for advice on specific provisions.

Sample Informed Consent

be removed. If agreed to, only that part of the ovary may be removed which in the opinion of the doctor is medically indicated. If my ovaries are removed during this procedure, I understand that I will experience premature menopause with its associated health impact including increased risk of heart disease and thinning of the bones (osteoporosis) and may require hormonal treatment. It is my understanding that ovaries left intact may have damage to their blood supply causing subsequent enlargement and pain and even ovarian failure. This condition may require additional surgery.

ADHESIONS. After any major abdominal operation some scar tissue (adhesions) may form and this may bind down the intestines and cause a subsequent intestinal obstruction (blocked bowels).

APPENDIX. If, in performing the surgical procedure, the doctor notices that the appendix has firm concretions (stone like masses) within, or there is evidence of previous inflammations or disease, I understand and agree that s/he (initial one of the following):

_____ may

_____ may not

perform an elective appendectomy. I understand that there is increased risk to me because of the chance of infection and the formation of scar tissue.

I have been told that the necessity for performing the total abdominal hysterectomy is because of:
_____
(describe in layman's terms)

I have been told that the alternatives of treatment include the following:
_____
_____
_____
_____

I have been advised of the risks involved with each of the above-listed alternative forms of treatment. The risks involved with NOT treating my condition are:
_____
_____

I have been advised that it is the opinion of my doctor that this operation is indicated and I have been given the opportunity of independent consultation prior to having this surgery.

I have been fully informed about the risks of a total abdominal hysterectomy and I am willing to undergo the operation. This does not relieve my doctor of any responsibilities for acts of negligence. I agree to undergo a total abdominal hysterectomy but expect that proper care shall be rendered to me at all times.

ANESTHESIA. I further understand that Dr. _____, the anesthesiologist, will give me full informed consent information about the alternative forms of anesthesia available and the risks of each form of anesthesia as it relates to me prior to the operation. Although my anesthesiologist will fully explain all the risks of anesthesia to me, I understand that with any operation or anesthesia there is a chance of death and/or brain damage from inadequate oxygen administered to me. I understand that if I have any form of spinal anesthesia, I may contract an infection, develop permanent paralysis secondary to bleeding and/or infection, as well as a temporary headache.

Signed:_____ Date:_____
(Patient or nearest relative)

_____
(Relationship)

Signed:_____ Date:_____
(Doctor)

Men Survey

Let's pretend you're visiting your doctor for your annual check up. Okay, okay—I know guys only go in for a check up every decade or so but PRETEND it's your ANNUAL check up. On top of that, let's pretend that you've been having difficulty urinating lately and that's what finally made you schedule the appointment.

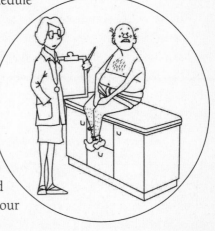

You're sitting on the edge of the examining table in your skivvies (and maybe your socks) and the doctor (let's say it's a female just for the heck of it—most women's docs are men so let's reverse it for the guys for the FULL effect of the question) anyway, your doctor tells you to drop your shorts and then proceeds to do an exam of your genitals.

When done, she tells you to pull up your shorts and then turns to make some notes on your chart. Then, in all seriousness, she turns back to you and says the following:

"You know John Doe Patient, you have an enlarged prostate gland. That's probably why you've been having difficulty urinating lately. I've reviewed your medical history and it's my recommendation that you undergo a procedure called HISterectomy—it's a procedure to surgically remove your testicles."

(Okay, the real name of the surgical procedure to remove a man's testicles is orchiectomy. For now, let's overlook the medical specifics and move on with the survey.)

Considering the doctor's recommendation, what do you do or say at this point?

The doctor proceeds with the discussion by saying the following:

"Well, I think you should know that you have a 75% chance of getting prostate cancer sometime in the next 10 years and we should really consider removing your testicles."

Now what do you do or say?

The doctor proceeds:

"You don't really plan on having any more children—right? So let's do this and remove the risk of cancer entirely. You do want to be around for your children as they're growing up, don't you?"

Now what do you do or say?

"John Doe Patient, a 75% chance of getting prostate cancer is very serious. I can schedule you for surgery within a week or two. Let's go ahead and set this up, okay?"

Now what do you do or say?

"John Doe Patient, you don't need to worry about the loss of testosterone—we have this terrific new patch you can wear that will give your body all the testosterone you need. Let's do this, okay? Believe me, your sexual life will NOT be impacted by this procedure."

Now what do you do or say?

Footnote

To put this in context for you so that you can have a better understanding of WHY I am asking these questions of men:

Nearly 600,000 women undergo hysterectomy annually. It has been speculated that as many as 90% of all hysterectomies—surgical removal of the uterus—are performed for benign conditions that are, in fact, treatable with methods that do not involve removal of the uterus at all.

According to the American College of Obstetricians and Gynecologists and as reported by the Center for Disease Control, only ~10% of all hysterectomies are due to cancer.

In addition, over 60% of the women who undergo hysterectomy have their ovaries removed at the same time. That's about 360,000 women or so annually. The ovaries perform an equivalent hormonal function of the testicles in a man.

Why do so many women readily allow this castration to happen to them? Because of one word: **cancer.** Doctors tell women that ovarian cancer—an incredibly deadly cancer—can be avoided entirely if they allow for the removal of their ovaries. What they DON'T tell women is astounding:

- The lifetime risk of acquiring ovarian cancer is 1.8%.
- If you undergo a hysterectomy (leaving the ovaries in), your risk factor is cut in half.
- Ovarian cancer can occur in the pelvic region even without the presence of the ovaries—if you're destined to get this type of cancer, removing the ovaries does not, necessarily, protect you.
- Removal of the ovaries means instant surgical menopause and a need for hormone replacement therapy (HRT) for the remainder of a woman's life. Without HRT, a woman's overall risk of acquiring heart disease and osteoporosis increases significantly. Heart disease is the number one killer of women in this nation.

During the last 20 years in the United States, over 12 million women have opted to have a hysterectomy under the guidance and advice of a gynecologist. Out of those 12 million, roughly 7.5 million women have consented to the removal of their ovaries at the same time. *7.5 million women castrated in the United States over the last 20 years for benign conditions of the uterus.*

So, compare how you responded with how women have responded under similar circumstances with significantly smaller statistical risk factors and ask yourself one question: Why?

When women say, "Not tonight dear, I have a headache." Could they possibly mean, "Not tonight dear, I have no sex drive and will get nothing out of this sexual encounter anyway so let's not. Okay?"

Cyberspace

Whether you own a computer or not, there simply couldn't be a better time than now to log on to the World Wide Web (WWW). How can you possibly do that if you don't own a computer? Well, if you haven't been to your local library lately, it's time to drop in, take a tour, and discover what's new. These days, most libraries have public access computers that are linked to the WWW. Even though I do happen to own a computer, whenever I'm traveling, I frequently drop into the local library to spend an hour or two getting caught up on my email.

Because the Internet connects your computer to a worldwide network of computers, you can share information with virtually anyone, almost anywhere, at any time of the day or night. The prospect of millions upon millions of individuals and computers all linked together and talking to one another at the same time is truly mind-boggling. To some, cyberspace technology is simply an overwhelming concept seemingly too difficult to figure out. Rest assured: You *are* capable of understanding the Internet! I hope that the information in this **Cyberspace** Appendix will help guide you through the process of logging on and using the Internet to seek out support from others as well as acquire medical information that will help educate and empower you to take charge of your health.

The Uterinefibroids email discussion group has members communicating with one another from all regions of the United States. It also has members from Canada, Japan, Singapore, Italy, Ireland, England, Australia, Norway, and regions of the Middle East and South Africa. Information can be transmitted and shared with others all over the world within a matter of minutes using the following:

➢ computer
➢ modem
➢ Internet Service Provider (ISP)
➢ web browser software (Netscape Navigator, Internet Explorer, AOL, etc.)

If you use a computer at the library, all these items are taken care of for you. In addition, most librarians are more than happy to take the time to show you how to use their equipment.

If you have a computer at home, it needs a modem—special telecommunications hardware installed inside your computer—to dial out to your ISP. An ISP is a business that has computers connected to the World Wide Web (WWW). When your computer modem dials into an ISP, that ISP then connects your computer to their computer. This connection is called a "handshake." If all is well and the ISP validates your password, then your computer connects to theirs. Their computer is the gateway to the WWW. Sort of like this:

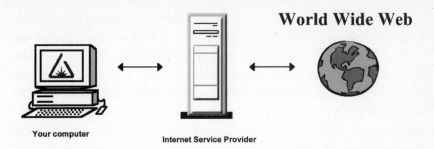

World Wide Web

Your computer

Internet Service Provider

When your computer "shakes hands" with your ISP's computer, you are literally shaking hands with the entire World Wide Web.

Once upon a time, a long time ago, a modem was a separate piece of hardware sitting next to your computer. Today, all new computers come with a modem already installed and ready to work for you. If yours doesn't, you'll need to visit the computer store to purchase one and have it installed.

To find an ISP, simply look in the yellow pages of your telephone directory under "Internet Services." Prices and services offered vary from one ISP to another, so don't hesitate to shop around. Also, don't be afraid to ask questions. If you're new to all this, tell them! Most ISPs are more than happy to help you and will take the necessary time to help you get connected to the WWW. On average, connecting to an ISP costs around $20/month. There are some ISPs that are free and yet others that cost as much as $100/month. Some ISPs allow for unlimited connection time and have local telephone numbers for you to use, but others limit the number of hours a month and, perhaps, use only a 1-800 number. In addition, cable television is getting into the act as technology moves forward with finding new ways to accommodate the millions of computers logging on to the WWW.

The final item you will need, in order to access the WWW, is web browser software. A web browser is a program that runs on your computer and allows you to send and receive email and visit websites. Computers sold today all come with a variety of web browsers already installed. If your computer doesn't have web browser software, rest assured that most ISPs will provide web browser software at no extra charge to you when you sign up for their services. The most popular web browsers today are Microsoft's Internet Explorer (IE) and Netscape's Navigator or Communicator. AOL (America Online) and CompuServe also provide their very own special web browsers as part of their connection services.

Your ISP will provide instructions that explain how to set up your web browser software with the correct phone numbers and how to dial into their service from your computer. These instructions vary from ISP to ISP and from web browser to web browser. Although it may seem complicated, it generally involves only typing in a telephone number, your ISP account name, and your ISP password. Furthermore, your computer will save this information for you so that it only has to be entered once. So, after you make it through the initial setup, you're home free! Well, almost. There are a few more things you need to know.

Email

Electronic mail (e-mail or email) allows you to send and receive messages whenever your computer is logged on to the WWW. Generally, your ISP supplies you with an email address that is unique to you, but you can also obtain additional email addresses for free at a number of websites on the WWW. These free email addresses allow you to send and receive email over the WWW with all that email stored on the email provider's computer. In addition, you can access these free email accounts from any computer logged on to the WWW without going through your own ISP first. For instance, when I'm visiting my mother (in another state), I can log on to the WWW using her computer and connecting to the WWW through her ISP, but then browse over to my free email account to check my email.

Free email accounts have an added benefit: they provide anonymity. You can create an email account using an entirely false name (pseudonym). Many women do not want to reveal their true identity to the entire world when discussing intensely personal medical situations. So, using a free email address can help you mask your identity. Even so, it is not okay to do things on the WWW that could be harmful to others or construed as a violation of the law while using a pseudonym email address. Rest assured, even pseudonym email addresses are traceable when slanderous email or illegal activities are involved.

There are many, many websites that offer free email addresses. To learn more about how you can obtain a free email address, the following is a short list of websites currently dedicated to this service.

Bigfoot
http://www.bigfoot.com

Eudoramail
http://www.eudoramail.com

Hotmail
http://www.hotmail.com

USA.Net Net@ddress
http://www.netaddress.com

URLs

URL (Unified Resource Locator) is the technical term for *web address*. The URL for the National Uterine Fibroids Foundation looks like this:

www.nuff.org

But, you might see the address also displayed like this:

http://www.nuff.org

The "http" stands for HyperText Transfer Protocol and represents one way in which information is transmitted over the WWW. Using most web browsers, you do NOT need to type in the "http://" portion of the web address (URL).

When you type in a URL, your web browser looks at it and then determines which computer to contact, which directory to review, and what specific page in that directory is the one you've requested. The web page is then delivered back to your web browser to display.

To understand how to read particularly long URLs, let's think in terms of a filing cabinet. Out on the WWW there are many, many filing cabinets. Let's say the web page you want looks like this:

http://www.4woman.gov/nwhic/references/dictionary.htm

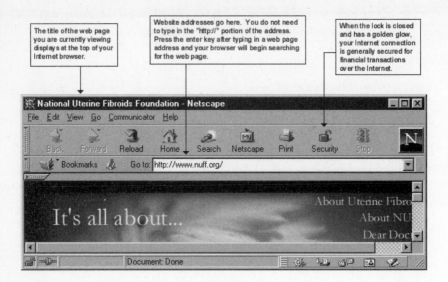

This is the web page address for the medical dictionary on the National Women's Health Information Center's (NWHIC) website. It's an awfully long web address, don't you think? Let's break it down. the first portion of this address is the actual primary address assigned to the NWHIC. It looks like this:

http://www.4women.gov

If you think of the WWW as a huge room filled with filing cabinets, then consider this portion of this address as only one of those cabinets.

This particular cabinet might have many drawers and one of those drawers might be labeled like this:

/nwhic

Inside of this drawer there are folders. Lots of them. The next part of the address is nothing more than a folder.

/references

(Indeed, this part of the address is a folder with a gateway web page entitled "Health Information for Special Groups.")

Inside that folder, there may be additional files. The final portion of the web address is the actual information page containing the content you are seeking. It represents the pages that might exist inside a file folder.

/dictionary.htm

Generally, files (actual web pages) end with **.htm** or **.html** or **.shtml**. The whole setup might look something like this:

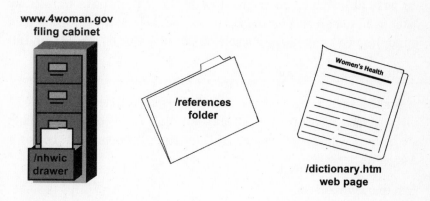

www.4woman.gov filing cabinet

/nhwic drawer

/references folder

Women's Health

/dictionary.htm web page

Of course, all this information is stored digitally on computers and not in actual hard paper format anywhere.

Because these addresses actually represent pages in a folder within a file drawer, it is quite common for web page owners to frequently re-arrange their pages and place them in a new folder or new file drawer. When they do this, those pages acquire a new address that includes the name of the new folder and new file drawer.

If, at any time, you attempt to locate a file and receive an error message instead, it's highly likely that the file was simply moved. You can always look at the URL and break it down to simply the main website address (the first section of the URL) and go there. Once there, you can generally search for the page you're looking for and locate it at its new address.

TIP: At the end of the main portion of every website address are let-ters that usually (but not always) represent a classification and/or loca-tion for the website. For instance, websites that end with **.org** are usually representative of nonprofit organizations, **.com** are commercial websites, **.edu** are educational websites, **.gov** are government websites, etc. A web-site ending with **.jp** might be located in Japan, and a website ending in **.uk** might be from England.

Searching

Over a billion web pages and growing every day. How in the world do you locate the web pages you need with that much information on the WWW? Well, never fear. The task has been simplified with search engines and search directories. My favorite search engine is called Google. With Google (as with all search engines), just type in a few descriptive words (like "uterine fibroids") and hit the Enter key (or click on the Google Search button), and a list of relevant results will display. Google can be found at:

http://www.google.com

Another search engine that I thoroughly enjoy is called Ask Jeeves. At this search engine, you ask a real question and a variety of search engines are queried with the results returned for you to choose from. Look for Ask Jeeves at:

http://www.ask.com

Perhaps one of the longest running and most popular search engines/directories on the WWW is Yahoo. At last count, there were twenty-one regional Yahoo search engines around the world—each one displayed in the native language of its region. The U.S. version can be found at:

http://www.yahoo.com

Search engines can also be found as an added feature on many websites. Typically, this allows you to search either the website or the entire WWW without actually leaving the website.

Creating a Bookmark Using Netscape Navigator

Bookmarking a web page is a way of storing URLs (web page addresses) on your own computer using your web browser software so that you can easily locate the page and return to it at a later time.

To create a bookmark for a web page:

1. Go to the web page on the WWW that you want to bookmark.
2. Click **Bookmarks.**

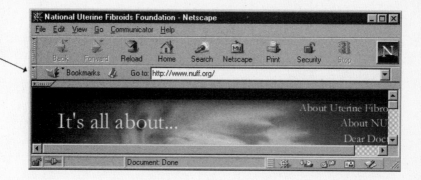

3. Choose Add Bookmark. The name of the web page is added to your Bookmark file.

To revisit a bookmarked web page:

1. Click **Bookmarks.**
2. Choose a bookmarked page from the menu and click on it.

Creating a Bookmark Using Internet Explorer

To create a bookmark for a web page:

1. Go to the web page on the WWW that you want to bookmark.
2. Click on **Favorites** folder.

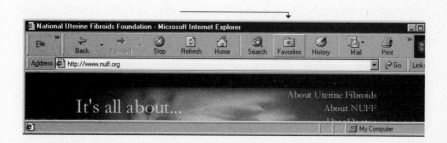

3. On the **Favorites** menu, click **Add to Favorites.**

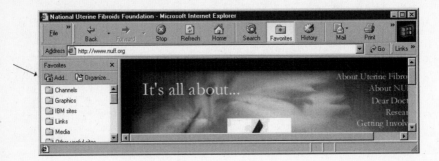

4. An **Add Favorite** box displays. Check for the **Name** of the website. At this point, you can type in a new name for the bookmarked website or you can leave it as is.

5. Click **OK** to bookmark the web page.

Tips

- To open one of your bookmarked pages, click the **Bookmarks** (Netscape) or **Favorites** folder (Microsoft Internet Explorer) and locate the desired web page. Click on its name.

- As your list of bookmarked web pages grows, you may want to organize them into folders.

Safety

Stalkers do exist on the WWW. People who mean you harm do exist on the WWW. People who would like nothing more than to take advantage of you in any way can and do exist on the WWW. Even so, it is possible to completely avoid troublesome encounters with these disturbed individuals.

First rule of thumb: Never post messages that contain your phone number or address. Sending email with this information to personal friends is okay—but sending it out over a discussion group can open you up to all sorts of unwanted correspondence. Think about the personal information you choose to share online very carefully before you actually post it.

Second rule of thumb: Delete all unsolicited email you receive immediately from your Inbox. Do not be tempted to click on the links in these messages and do not respond in any way, shape, or form. Specifically, do not even send back a message saying you want to be removed from their mailing list. Why not? Because when you do so, you confirm your email address for them. Not only will you not be removed from their mailing list, but your email address will also be sold to others.

Third rule of thumb: Stay off pornography websites. Don't even be remotely tempted to go there. Many of these sites have hidden costs and do a "phone-line switch" on you that may result in hundreds of dollars getting charged to your long distance phone bill. On top of that, you become a "target" for solicitation and may find yourself inundated with pornographic email.

Final rule of thumb: If you receive an email from someone you do not know, do not open any attachment that may be connected to it. In fact, delete it immediately and then empty your email trash folder. Viruses are commonly sent as email attachments. It doesn't hurt to be suspicious of *all* attachments that come with incoming email. Do not open an attachment unless there is a reasonable explanation for it included in the email message you receive. When in doubt, email the individual and ask if an attachment was sent or not and, if so, what was it supposed to be? Some viruses work on an individual's computer without the individual even knowing about it. Every time an email is sent—*violà*—the virus is attached.

Medical Information on the Internet

Not all the information on the WWW is accurate. It is critical for you to research what you learn and not blindly accept an individual's word as authority. It's also extremely important to not act on any medical information you find on the Internet without having a detailed discussion with your physician first. The Bibliography of this book provides an excellent starting point for you to begin your research on the WWW. The websites listed are reputable and reliable. Even so, medical information is constantly changing and web pages may or may not be kept up to reflect those changes. Medical disclaimers exist on these websites for a very real reason: the individuals and organizations providing medical information on the WWW want you to talk to your doctor! Indeed, you should. The WWW is a *research* and *support group* and *communication* tool. *It is **not** a physician.*

Discussion Groups

Discussion groups are the WWW's way of providing active, ongoing communication with large groups of individuals all interested in the same subject matter. Typically, there is a web page associated with each discussion group that explains the purpose of the group and provides instructions on how you can participate. Some discussion groups are handled entirely through email. Others are message boards: places where you type in your response and when you click the Submit button, it displays your response on the website for others to read. Some discussion groups have restricted access and are password protected, while others are open for everyone on the WWW to participate in and read.

Medical or health-related groups make up a major portion of discussion groups on the WWW. Just about every disease or medical condition known today probably already has a discussion group dedicated to discussing the issues or serving as a support group for members who suffer from the condition. A current list of the most popular women's health groups can be found on pages 292 through 303. In addition, an updated list can be found at www.uterinefibroids.com.

Netiquette

Rules of good behavior and consideration for others are expected on the WWW just as they are in your own home. The term **Netiquette** was coined to refer directly to Internet etiquette—rules of expected behavior. Most email and bulletin board discussion groups have their own set of rules for members to follow, and it's usually a good idea to take the time to read these rules *before* you begin posting your own messages. Whenever you bring together a few hundred people online participating in a single discussion group, rules are definitely necessary! Here are a few basic starter rules that most groups follow:

1. Do not type your messages in all capital letters. THIS IS CONSID-
ERED SHOUTING!
2. Junk mail (unsolicited email from people you don't know) on the
WWW is called spam. Most people do NOT appreciate spam. Do not
use any medical support group or message board as a tool to sell your
products or services.
3. Do not forward every piece of amusing email or every computer virus
warning you receive to everyone you know. Doing this clogs up the
WWW with massive quantities of unnecessary email and can even
crash computers by overloading them. Be thoughtful and selective in
what you choose to forward to others.
4. Be aware that on email discussion groups your email may be read by
hundreds of individuals and may also be archived, or stored, online
for a very long time. Think before you type and think again before
you hit the Send button.
5. Try to develop an understanding of the difference between thoughtful
analysis and negative criticism. Thoughtful analysis can include negative commentary but doesn't usually contain personal attacks. Negative criticisms meant to personally hurt another are never appreciated
and can even get your permanently barred from a discussion group.

Final Thoughts

Although it's easy to think of computers as nothing more than inanimate
objects incapable of emotions, the truth is they can bring to your Inbox a
pile of email filled with love, hate, anger, frustration, surprise, and even
comic relief. It doesn't take long for your computer to become an exten-
sion of who you are and to bring along with it a wide range of emotions
for all the people you encounter on your journeys around the WWW. In
addition, medical information you discover online can be devastating or,
quite incredibly, save your life. The emotions tied to what you may discover online can also make your computer a very real lifeline to the outside world. Within this 'virtual' world, you may find yourself seeking
support from individuals you've never met and you can't even see or
touch. They may even live in another country halfway around the world.

It certainly seems surreal and quite impossible at times, but some of
my best friends today are women and men I've met over the WWW. In

my most isolated moments of deep despair and poor health, women came online to touch my heart and changed me forever. The power of the WWW is quickly transferred to each person who logs on to this incredibly well networked, virtual information beast I like to call **Cyberspace.**

A very long time ago, my grandmother taught me that when a visitor knocks on your door at dinnertime, there's always room for one more place setting at the table. Who would've ever thought that this adage would apply so poignantly to the World Wide Web? But it does. Please join us. *There's always room for one more. . . .* ☺

Commonly Used WWW Acronyms

AAMOF	as a matter of fact
BBFN	bye bye for now
BFN	bye for now
BTW	by the way
BYKT	but you knew that
CMIIW	correct me if I'm wrong
EOL	end of lecture
FAQ	frequently asked question(s)
FITB	fill in the blank
FWIW	for what it's worth
FYI	for your information
HTH	hope this helps
IAC	in any case
IAE	in any event
IMCO	in my considered opinion
IMHO	in my humble opinion
IMNSHO	in my not so humble opinion
IMO	in my opinion
IOW	in other words
LOL	laughing out loud
MHOTY	my hat's off to you
NRN	no reply necessary
OIC	oh, I see
OTOH	on the other hand
ROF	rolling on the floor
ROFL	rolling on the floor laughing

RSN	real soon now
SITD	still in the dark
TIA	thanks in advance
TIC	tongue in cheek
TTFN	Ta-ta for now
TTYL	talk to you later
TYVM	thank you very much
WYSIWYG	what you see is what you get
<G>	Grinning
<J>	Joking
<L>	Laughing
<S> or :)	Smiling
:þ	Sticking Tongue Out
;)	Winking
<Y>	Yawning

Glossary

Abdomen The part of the body below the ribs and above the pelvis.

ACOG Abbreviation for American College of Obstetricians and Gynecologists; professional member-based organization for obstetricians and gynecologists.

Adeno Abbreviation for adenomyosis.

Adenomatous hyperplasia Excessive cell growth in the endometrial lining of the uterus.

Adenomyosis Tissue similar to endometriosis found between the muscle fibers in the wall of the uterus.

Adhesion Abnormal tissue growth, typically developing after surgery and sticking together; internal scar tissue.

Adrenals Glands located on top of the kidneys that produce hormones such as testosterone and estrogen.

Amenorrhea Lack of menstruation.

Analgesic Pain-relieving drug.

Anastomoses The connection of separate blood vessels resulting in a shared blood flow.

Anemia A reduction in red blood cells resulting in inadequate oxygen flow to tissue and organs; often the result of prolonged and abnormal menstrual bleeding.

Anesthesia Pain relief medication.

Angiogram An x-ray of one or more blood vessels produced by angiography.

Anovulate Failure to ovulate; when an egg is not released from either ovary.

Asymptomatic Without symptoms.

Atrophic vaginitis Vaginal dryness typically due to absence of estrogen.

Atrophy Drying up of tissue.

Atypical hyperplasia Abnormal cell proliferation; in the female reproductive system, a precancerous condition of the endometrium. Hyperplasia with atypia.

Benign Not cancer (noncancerous).

Bilateral salpingo-oophorectomy The removal of both fallopian tubes and both ovaries.

Biopsy A surgical procedure during which a small tissue specimen is removed and examined for the presence of disease.

Bladder A sac-like organ in the pelvic region where urine is stored before it leaves the body.

Board certification An indication that the physician has completed additional specialized training and passed an examination.

Bookmark Marking and storing URLs (web page addresses) using a computer's web browser software.

Breakthrough bleeding Unscheduled/irregular uterine bleeding.

Cancer A disease of the body's cells; cells become abnormal and grow out of control, even spreading to other parts of the body.

Castration Removal of the ovaries or testes.

Catheter A hollow, flexible tube for insertion into a body opening or blood vessel to allow the passage of fluids or to open a passageway. A catheter may be used for the drainage of urine from the bladder through the urethra or insertion through a blood vessel for diagnostic or procedural purposes.

Cervical canal Area from vagina through the cervix to the body of the uterus.

Cervical dysplasia Abnormal cell changes on the cervix. May progress to cancer.

Cervix The lower portion of the uterus.

Chromosome The self-replicating structure of cells containing the DNA that carries in its composition the specific arrangement of genes.

Chronic condition A condition that lasts or keeps coming back over a long period of time.

Colposcopy An examination of the vagina and cervix using a special microscope.

Cone biopsy A surgical procedure where a cone-shaped section of the cervix is removed for diagnostic purposes.

Constipation Irregular and infrequent or difficult evacuation of the bowels.

Chronic endometritis Inflammation of the endometrium that occurs frequently or lasts a long period of time.

Compassionate use A situation where a drug is provided to a patient on humanitarian grounds prior to FDA approval of the drug. Typically allowed in life threatening situations where the drug is still undergoing testing for efficacy but the patient has limited treatment options.

Cryoablation The removal of the endometrium through a freezing process.

Cryomyolysis The destruction of blood flow in uterine fibroids through a freezing process.

Cyberspace World Wide Web. The electronic world of computer networks, in which online communication takes place.

Cystocele A condition where part of the bladder protrudes/drops into the vagina.

Cystourethrocele Combination of the bladder and urethra protruding/dropping into the vagina.

D&C (dilation and curettage) A surgical procedure that involves dilating (opening) the cervix and scraping the uterine lining (endometrium).

Dysmenorrhea Painful menstrual cramps.

Dyspareunia Painful sexual intercourse.

Dysplasia The growth of abnormal cells. Dysplasia is a precancerous condition that may or may not turn into cancer at a later time.

Email Mail sent and received electronically through the use of computers.

Embolization The introduction of a substance into a blood vessel to stop bleeding or to treat abnormal blood vessels or tumors.

Endo Abbreviation for endometriosis.

Endocrinology The study of hormones.

Endometrial ablation A surgical procedure in which lasers and electrical currents are used to remove the endometrium.

Endometrial biopsy A sample of endometrial tissue is removed and examined for abnormal cells. See biopsy.

Endometrioma Endometrial tissue growing in an ovary.

Endometriosis A condition in which tissue that lines the walls of the uterus migrates and grows outside the uterus; implanting itself elsewhere in the pelvic cavity.

Endometrium The tissue that lines the inside of the uterus.

Endoscope A special instrument used in the visual examination of the interior of a bodily canal or a hollow organ.

Endoscopy Visual examination of the interior of a bodily canal or a hollow organ using an endoscope.

Enterocele A loop of intestine protrudes/drops between the rectum and vagina.

Estradiol The strongest form of estrogen produced by the ovaries.

Estrogen A hormone produced in the ovaries that affects the growth and health of female reproductive functions and organs.

Fallopian tubes Tubes located on either side of the uterus that eggs travel through when they move from the ovary to the uterus.

FDA Abbreviation for Food and Drug Administration.

Female reconstructive surgery Term coined by Vicki Hufnagel to represent a wide range of corrective female gynecological procedures performed during one operation.

Femoral hematoma A swelling of blood from the femoral artery, the primary artery of the thigh.

Fibro Abbreviation for fibromyalgia.

Fibroids Benign (noncancerous) tumors that grow on the inside of the uterus, within the wall of the uterus and/or on its outer surface.

Fibroma Uterine fibroid.

Fibromyalgia A condition with symptoms of muscle pain, stiffness and fatigue. Cause unknown.

Fibromyoma Uterine fibroid.

Follicle A tiny bubble in which each egg in the ovary develops.

Follicle-stimulating hormone Hormone released by the pituitary to stimulate maturation of follicles.

Food and Drug Administration United States government agency that oversees and approves the use of drugs and medical devices (as well as all food products).

FSH Abbreviation for follicle-stimulating hormone.

Fundus The top of the uterus; the area between the fallopian tubes.

Gastrointestinal Relating to or affecting both the stomach and intestines.

Genetic Inherited, as with genes; tending to occur among members of a family usually by heredity.

GnRH Abbreviation for gonadotropin-releasing hormone.

Gonadotropin-releasing hormone (GnRH) A hormone released by the hypothalamus that tells the pituitary to release follicle-stimulating hormones (FSH) and luteinizing hormones (LH) in order to get the menstrual cycle going each month. Synthetically, this is an anti-estrogen hormone sometimes prescribed to shrink fibroid tumors (off-label). More typically prescribed (on-label) to reduce abnormal bleeding and allow a patient to improve her hematocrit prior to surgery.

Hematocrit The ratio of the volume of packed red blood cells to the volume of whole blood.

Hemoglobin The iron-containing protein pigment in red blood cells that carries oxygen from the lungs to the tissues and organs of the body.

Hemorrhage Uncontrolled bleeding.

Hemorrhoids Swelling of the anus and lower part of the rectum caused by an expansion of the blood vessels and resulting in a bloody or mucus discharge.

Hormone A chemical produced by the body that regulates certain bodily functions; synthetic (man-made) hormones are used in birth control pills and in medicines to treat certain conditions.

Hormone replacement therapy Manufactured chemicals, using either natural or synthetically produced compounds, meant to replace or supplement the natural hormones a woman's body produces.

Hot flashes Intense feelings of heat throughout the body that occur during menopause in response to diminished estrogen or during treatment with drugs that block estrogen production.

HRT Abbreviation for hormone replace therapy.

HTTP Abbreviation for hypertext transfer protocol.

Hydronephrosis An accumulation of urine in the kidney, typically as a result of obstruction in the urinary passages.

Hyperplasia An overgrowth of the uterine lining, probably caused by excess estrogen. This is sometimes considered to be a precancerous condition, particularly in women who are near or through menopause.

Hypertext transfer protocol A protocol for transfering hypertext requests and information between computer servers and browsers.

Hypoactive sexual desire disorder Abnormally lacking in a desire for sex.

Hypothalamus A hormone producing gland in the brain that initiates the menstrual cycle.

Hypothyroidism A medical disorder resulting from insufficient production of thyroid.

Hysterectomy Surgical removal of the uterus. Sometimes, the cervix and/or ovaries and fallopian tubes are also removed.

Hysterosalpinogography (HSG) A procedure in which a small amount of fluid is injected in to the uterus and fallopian tubes to determine whether the tubes are blocked or if there are any abnormal changes in size or shape of the uterus or tubes.

Hysteroscope A thin, lighted tube that is inserted into the vagina to examine the cervix and inside of the uterus.

Hysteroscopic myomectomy Vaginal removal of submucosal fibroids with the use of a hysterscope.

Hysteroscopy An examination of the inside of the uterus using a hysteroscope.

Hysterosonogram The injection of a small amount of water into the uterine cavity so that the lining of the uterus is more clearly defined during a transvaginal ultrasound.

IBS Abbreviation for irritable bowel syndrome.

IC Abbreviation for interstitial cystitis.

Incision Surgical cut.

Infertility Inability to conceive and/or complete a successful pregnancy after twelve months of intercourse without the use of any form of birth control.

Informed consent The concept of informing and educating a patient considering surgery on the surgical risks, benefits, and alternative forms of treatment prior to actually agreeing to the surgery.

Internet A network of computers connected around the world that allows for the exchange of information.

Internet service provider A company which provides other companies or individuals the access to a network connection used to link one computer to another and to allow access to the WWW of information.

Interstitial cystitis A bladder inflammation.

Intramural fibroids Benign tumor that grows within the myometrium or uterine wall.

Irritable bowel syndrome Recurrent abdominal pain and diarrhea frequently alternating with periods of constipation and possibly associated with emotional stress.

Junk mail Unsolicited, unwanted email from people you don't know. Spam.

Kegel exercises Special exercises to tighten the pelvic muscles. These exercises are one method used to treat uterine prolapse and urinary incontinence (losing urine when you don't want to) as well as bowel control.

LAH Abbreviation for laparoscopic assisted hysterectomy.

Lap Abbreviation for laparoscope or laparoscopy.

Laparoscope A slender, light-transmitting instrument that is used to view the pelvic organs or perform surgery.

Laparoscopic assisted hysterectomy Removal of the entire uterus (including the cervix) abdominally with the use of a laparoscope.

Laparoscopic assisted vaginal hysterectomy Removal of the entire uterus (including the cervix) vaginally with the assisted use of a laparoscope.

Laparoscopic assisted vaginal myomectomy Vaginal removal of fibroids with the assisted use of a laparoscope.

Laparoscopic myomectomy Abdominal removal of fibroids with the use of a laparoscope.

Laparoscopic supracervical hysterectomy Removal of the upper portion of the uterus (leaving the cervix intact) abdominally through the use of a laparascope.

Laparoscopy A procedure that allows the doctor to look inside the pelvic cavity or perform surgery by inserting a tube-like instrument through a small cut in the abdomen.

Laparotomy Abdominal surgical procedure; a form of myomectomy to remove uterine fibroids.

LAVH Abbreviation for laparoscopic assisted vaginal hysterectomy.

Leiomyoma The medical term for a fibroid tumor.

Leiomyosarcoma Cancerous tumor of the uterus.

LH Abbreviation for luteinizing hormone.

Ligaments A band of tissue that can stretch and that supports other parts of the body.

LSH Abbreviation for laparoscopic supracervical hysterectomy.

Luteinizing hormone A hormone from the pituitary gland that stimulates the release of progesterone.

Magnetic resonance imaging Diagnostic test that uses a high-power magnet and a computer to gain images of internal body tissues.

Malignant Cancerous.

Menopause "The change"; the time when a woman's ovaries stop producing estrogen and discontinue releasing eggs; menstruation stops.

Menorrhagia Abnormally heavy menstrual flow.

Menstrual cycle The four-week period each month when an egg develops in the ovary, the lining of the uterus thickens, and the egg is released. If the egg is not fertilized, the cycle is completed when the lining of the uterus is shed through menstruation (a woman's "period").

Menstruation The shedding of the lining of the uterus that occurs each month when a woman does not become pregnant; commonly referred to as a woman's "period."

Mifepristone A drug which blocks the body's use of progesterone. Taken orally to induce abortion but currently also under investigation as a potential treatment for uterine fibroids.

Misembolization The process in which an unintended blood vessel or organ is obstructed by the placement of embolic materials.

Modem A device used in the transmission of digital information using the telephone. The piece of computer equipment (usually located inside the hardware server box) that connects a computer to the internet through telephone lines.

MRI Abbreviation for magnetic resonance imaging; diagnostic test that uses a high-power magnet and a computer to gain images of internal body tissues.

Musculoskeletal Relating to or involving the muscles and the skeleton (bones).

Myofibroma Uterine fibroid.

Myolysis A surgical procedure in which instruments are inserted through tiny, laparoscopic incisions in the abdomen and, using a special probe, a high frequency electrical current is sent to the fibroid, thereby destroying its blood supply.

Myoma Uterine fibroid.

Myomectomy A surgical procedure to remove fibroid tumors.

Myometrium Muscular wall of the uterus.

Natural hormone replacement therapy Compounded hormone formulas, using or related to natural food products, meant to replace or supplement the hormones a woman's body produces; for example, progesterone cream.

Naturopathic Therapy that relies on natural remedies, such as diet and combinations of herbs and vitamins, to treat illness.

Netiquette Internet etiquette; conventions of politeness recognized on email list groups and message boards on the WWW.

NHRT Abbreviation for natural hormone replacement therapy.

Off-label Use of an FDA approved medical drug or device in a manner that is not specifically indicated on the label. Typically, clinical testing requirements have not been met and reviewed by the FDA for the specific use of the product as its being prescribed/used.

On-label Use of an FDA approved medical drug or device precisely as indicated on the manufacturing label; clinical testing requirements have been met and reviewed by the FDA for indicated uses and subsequently approved by the FDA.

Oophorectomy Surgical removal of an ovary.

Orchiectomy Surgical removal of one or both testes.

Orgasmic disorder Persistent or recurrent difficulty, delay in, or absence of, attaining orgasm following sufficient sexual stimulation and arousal causing personal distress.

Ovarian cancer Malignant tumor of the ovary. Number one cause of death from gynecologic cancers.

Ovarian cyst The formation of a fluid filled sac on the surface of the ovary each month after an egg is released from the ovary during normal ovulation. Large cysts can cause pain and even rupture, causing bleeding.

Ovary Small organ, located on either side of the uterus, that contains eggs and produces hormones, such as estrogens.

Pain mapping The process of pinpointing the source of pain to determine appropriate medical treatment by logging occurrences, undergoing corresponding diagnostic tests and, through a process of elimination, identifying the source of pain.

Pap smear A procedure in which cells are removed from the cervix during a vaginal exam, placed on a slide, and examined through a microscope to look for cancer or precancerous conditions.

PCA Abbreviation for patient controlled administration; generally used in reference to a machine that allows the patient to control the dosaging of anesthetics, such as morphine, through an intravenous line.

Pedunculated submucosal fibroid Benign tumor that grows from the endrometrium and hangs down into the uterine cavity from a stalk.

Pedunculated subserosal fibroid Benign tumor that grows from a stalk on the outer wall of the uterus.

Pelvic exam Examination of the internal and external reproductive organs.

Perimenopause Transition from reproductive to nonreproductive (hormonal) status.

Pfannensteil Horizontal abdominal incision placed just above the pubic hairline and named after Dr. Herman Johann Pfannensteil, the physician recognized as having first used this incision to reduce morbidity and speed recovery in obese patients. Bikini cut.

PID Abbreviation for product insert datasheet; information brochure that accompanies drugs and devices.

Polyps Benign (noncancerous) growths that develop from the endometrial lining.

Polyvinyl alcohol Also called PVA; embolic material used in uterine artery embolization.

Progesterone A hormone produced in the ovaries that prepares the lining of the uterus (endometrium) to receive a fertilized egg. When progesterone levels decrease, menstruation occurs.

Prolapse To fall or drop, as a uterus or bladder might if the ligaments holding it in place become stretched.

Prostate Related to the prostate gland; a gland surrounding the urethra at the base of a man's bladder that produces a fluid which is a component of semen.

PVA Abbreviation for polyvinyl alcohol particles.

Rapidly growing fibroid Any fibroid that grows and causes the uterus to increase in gestational size of six weeks or more during the course of an entire year.

Rectocele A condition whereby the wall of the rectum protrudes into the vagina.

Rectum The bottom portion of the large intestine.

Reproductive system The organs of the body that allow a woman to become pregnant and carry and give birth to a child; includes the uterus, fallopian tubes, ovaries, and vagina.

Resectoscope A slender telescope with an electrical wire loop or rollerball tip used to remove or destroy tissue inside the uterus.

Salpingo-oophorectomy Removal of the ovary and fallopian tube.

Search engine A program or database that allows keyword searches for information on the Internet.

Sexual arousal disorder Persistent or recurring inability to attain, or to maintain sufficient sexual excitement thereby causing personal distress.

Sexual aversion disorder Persistent or recurring phobic aversion to, and avoidance of, sexual contact with a sexual partner, which causes personal distress.

SH Abbreviation for supracervical hysterectomy (abdominal).

Sonogram An imaging procedure in which echoes from sound waves passing through tissues create pictures of structures deep within the body.

Spam Unsolicited electronic mail sent indiscriminately to multiple mailing lists, individuals, message boards, or newsgroups.

Speculum A metal or plastic instrument the doctor inserts into the vagina to help examine the vagina and cervix.

Sterilization Surgical procedure that makes reproduction (pregnancy) no longer possible.

Submucosal fibroid Benign tumor that grows and protrudes into the endometrial cavity of the uterus.

Subserosal fibroid Benign tumor that grows from the serosal surface (outer portion) of the uterus.

Supracervical hysterectomy (abdominal) Removal of the uterus through the abdomen with the retention of the cervix.

Symptomatic Having symptoms, typically in reference to illness or disease.

TAH Abbreviation for total abdominal hysterectomy.

TAH/BSO Abbreviation for total abdominal hysterectomy with bilateral salpingo oophorectomy.

Thyroid stimulating hormone A hormone released by the pituitary that activates production and release of thyroid hormones.

Total abdominal hysterectomy Removal of the entire uterus (including the cervix) through an abdominal incision.

Total abdominal hysterectomy with bilateral salpingo-oophorectomy Removal of the entire uterus (including the cervix), ovaries and fallopian tubes through an abdominal incision.

Total vaginal hysterectomy Removal of the entire uterus (including the cervix) through the vagina.

Transabdominal ultrasound Diagnostic test involving a hand-held instrument placed over the abdomen and used to send sound waves to internal organs which are then visualized on a video monitor. See ultrasound or sonogram.

Transvaginal ultrasound An ultrasound that includes the insertion of a probe into the vagina.

TSH Abbreviation for thyroid stimulating hormone.

TVH Abbreviation for total vaginal hysterectomy.

UAE Abbreviation for uterine artery embolization.

UFE Abbreviation for uterine fibroid embolization.

Ultrasound Diagnostic test where sound waves are used to "view" internal structures.

Unilateral salpingo oophorectomy Surgical removal of one ovary.

Urethrocele A prolapse condition where the urethra protrudes/drops into the vagina.

Urinary incontinence Inability to hold urine.

URL Abbreviation for uniform resource locator; unique address identifier for websites.

Urologic Pertaining to the urinary tract or urology.

USO Abbreviation for unilateral salpingo oophorectomy.

Uterine artery embolization Use of interventional materials to stop the blood flow in the uterine artery feeding uterine fibroids.

Uterine fibroid Benign (noncancerous) tumor that grows on the inside of the uterus, within the wall of the uterus and/or on its outer surface.

Uterine fibroid embolization See uterine artery embolization.

Uterus Muscular organ located in the pelvis capable of containing and nourishing a developing embryo and fetus during pregnancy; womb; the normal site of implantation of fertilized eggs.

Vagina Area or passage from the uterus to the genitals.

Vaginismus A painful contraction or spasm of the vagina.

Virus (computer) A computer program that is designed to have a negative effect on a computer's memory or machine coding.

von Willebrand Disease A bleeding disorder. For more information, call the National Hemophilia Foundation 1-800-424-2634.

Watchful waiting The doctor sees the patient regularly to keep track of the condition and typically attempts symptom relief through non-invasive measures.

web browser A software program used to access and view web pages over the WWW.

Womb Uterus.

World Wide Web A collection of internet websites accessible through hypertext transfer protocol (HTTP).

WWW Abbreviation for World Wide Web.

Bibliography/References

Introduction

Broder, MS, Kanouse, DE, Mittman, BS, Bernstein, SJ. "The Appropriateness of Recommendations for Hysterectomy" *Obstet Gynec* 2000;95(2):199–205.

Lepine, LA, Hillis, SD, Marchbanks, PA, Koonin, LM, Morrow, B, Kieke, BA, Wilcox, LS. "Hysterectomy Surveillance—United States, 1980–1993." *Morbidity and Mortality Weekly Report* 1997;46(SS-4):1–15.

National Center for Health Statistics. "Ambulatory and Inpatient Procedures in the United States, 1996." Hyattsville, Maryland: Public Health Service, 1998; DHHS Publication No. (PHS) 99–1710.

Chapter 1 Why Me?

Center for Disease Control and Prevention, *Fastats A to Z,* http://www.cdc.gov/nchs/fastats/women.htm, 7/13/99.

Chiaffarino, F, Parazzini, F, La Vecchia, C, Chatenoud, L, De Cintio, E, Marsico, S. "Diet and Uterine Myomas." *Obstet Gynec* 1999;94(3):395–398.

Chapter 2 Anatomy of a Fibroid

American College of Obstetricians & Gynecologists. *Hysteroscopy*. Patient Education Pamphlet, 1992.

American College of Obstetricians & Gynecologists. *Laparoscopy*. Patient Education Pamphlet, 1996.

American College of Obstetricians & Gynecologists. *Uterine Fibroids*. Patient Education Pamphlet, 1999.

American College of Obstetricians & Gynecologists. *Uterine Leiomyomata*. Technical Bulletin 1994;192:863–870.

Burroughs, KD. "The Role of Ovarian Hormones in the Development and Growth of Uterine Leiomyoma." Dissertation. The University of Texas at Austin, December 1998.

Buttram, V, Jr., Reiter, R. "Uterine Leiomyomata: Etiology, Symptomatology, and Management." *Fertility and Sterility* 1981;36(4):433–445.

Cramer, DW. "Epidemiology of Myomas." *Sem In Repro Endocrinol* 1992;10:320–24.

Cramer, SF, Patel, A. "The Frequency of Uterine Leiomyomas." *Am J Clin Pathol* 1990;94(4):435–438.

Institute for Clinical Systems Improvement (ICSI). "Diagnosis and Management of Infertility." 1999

Kjerulff, KH, Langenberg, P, Seidman, JD, Stolley, PD, Guzinski, GM. "Uterine Leiomyomas: Racial Differences in Severity, Symptoms and Age at Diagnosis." *J Reprod Med* 1996;41:483–490.

Marshall, LM, Spiegelman, D, Barbieri, RL, Goldman, MB, et al. "Variation in the Incidence of Uterine Leiomyoma among Premenopausal Women by Age and Race." *Obstet Gynecol* 1997;90:967–973.

Montague, A, Swartz, DP, Woodruff, JD. "Sarcoma Arising in Leiomyoma of Uterus: Factors influencing Prognosis." *Am J Obstet Gynecol* 1965;92:421.

Parker, W, Fu, Y, Berek, J. "Uterine Sarcoma in Patients Operated on for Presumed Leiomyoma and Rapidly Growing Leiomyoma." *Obstet Gynecol* 1994;83:414–18.

Ries, LAG, Kosary, CL, Hankey, BF, Miller, BA, Clegg, L, Edwards, BK, eds. *SEER Cancer Statistics Review, 1973–1996*. Bethesday, MD: National Cancer Institute, 1999.

Samadi, AR, Lee, NC, Flanders, WD, Boring, JR, III, Parris, EB. "Risk Factors for Self-Reported Uterine Fibroids: A Case-Control Study." *Am J Public Health* 1996;86:858–862.

Sampson, JA. "The Blood Supply of Uterine Myomata." *Surgery, Gynecology and Obstetrics* 1912;14:215–230.

Chapter 3 The Choices

Angell, M. "Is Academic Medicine for Sale?" Editorial. *NEJM* 2000;342(20): 1516–1518. http://www.nejm.org/content/2000/0342/0020/1516.asp

Bernhardt, SA, McCulley, GA. "Knowledge Management and Pharmaceutical Development Teams: Using Writing to Guide Science." *Technical Communication: IEEE Transactions on Professional Communication* February/March 2000;47(1):22–34.

Bodenheimer, T. "Uneasy Alliance—Clinical Investigators and the Pharmaceutical Industry." NEJM 2000;342(20):1539–1544. http://www.nejm.org/content/2000/0342/0020/1539.asp

Food and Drug Administration, Department of Health and Human Services. "Medical Devices; Current Good Manufacturing Practice (CGMP) Final Rule; Quality System Regulation." *Federal Register:* October 7, 1996;61(195):52601–52662. http://www.fda.gov/cdrh.

Greenberg, MD, Kazamel, TIG. "Medical and Socioeconomic Impact of Uterine Fibroids." *Obstet and Gyn Clinics of North America* 1995;22(4):625–636.

IMS America, Ltd. "Pediatric Drug Studies: Protecting Pint-Sized Patients." *FDA Consumer Magazine* May–June 1999. http://www.fda.gov/fdac/features/1999/399_kids.html#chart

Marks, NF, Shinberg, DS. "Socioeconomic Differences in Hysterectomy: The Wisconsin Longitudinal Study." *American Journal of Public Health* 1997;87(9):1507–1515.

Natural Health Village. *Alternative Medicine: Expanding Medical Horizons: A Report to the National Institutes of Health on Alternative Medical Systems and Practices in the United States.* Prepared under the auspices of the Workshop on Alternative Medicine, Chantilly, Virginia, September 14–16, 1992.

Ries, LAG, Kosary, CL, Hankey, BF, Miller, BA, Clegg, L, Edwards, BK, eds. *SEER Cancer Statistics Review,* 1973–1996. Bethesda, MD: National Cancer Institute, 1999.

Thakar, R, Manyonda, I. "Total Versus Subtotal Hysterectomy: A Survey of Current Views and Practice Among British Gynecologists." *Journal of Obstetrics & Gynaecology,* May 1998; 18(3)267–269.

Virtanen, HS, Makinen, JI, Kiilholma, PJA. "Conserving the Cervix at Hysterectomy." *British Journal of Obstetrics and Gynaecology* 1995;102:587.

Wood, AJ, Stein, CM, Woosley, R. "Making Medicines Safer—The Need for an Independent Drug Safety Board." *N Engl J Med* 1998;339(25):1851–4.

Zimmerman, BB, Schultz, JR. "A Study of the Effectiveness of Information Design Principles Applied to Clinical Research Questionnaires." *Technical Communication* May 2000;47(2):177–194.

Chapter 4 Ignore the Fibroids

Edwards, S. "Women Who Have Undergone a Tubal Sterilization Have a Reduced Risk of Contracting Ovarian Cancer." *Family Planning Perspectives* 1994;26(2):90–91.

Hollander, D. "Risk of Ovarian Cancer Is Lessened by Childbearing Pill Use and Hysterectomy." *Family Planning Perspectives* 1995;(27)(2):94–95.

Chapter 5 Treat the Symptoms

American College of Obstetricians & Gynecologists. *Abnormal Uterine Bleeding.* Patient Education Pamphlet, 1999.

Gladwell, Malcolm. "John Rock's Error: What the Co-Inventor of the Pill Didn't Know: Menstruation Can Endanger Women's Health." *The New Yorker,* March 13, 2000; 52–63.

Goldfarb, HA. "A Review of 35 Endometrial Ablations Using the Nd:YAG Laser for Recurrent Menometrorrhagia." *Obstet Gynecol* 1990;76(5):833–835.

Grady, H. "Immunomodulation Through Castor Oil Packs." *Journal of Naturopathic Medicine* 1999; 7(1).

Hammond, CB. *Confronting Aging and Disease: The Role of HRT.* Women's Health Treatment Updates. Medical Education Collaborative, 1999. http://www.medscape.com/Medscape/WomensHealth/TreatmentUpdate/1999/tu01/public/toc-tu01.html

Lobo, RA. "Menopause Management for the Millennium." *Women's Health Clinical Management Volume 1.* Medical Education Collaborative, 1999. http://www.medscape.com/Medscape/WomensHealth/ClinicalMgmt/CM.v01/public/index.CM.v01.html

MotherNature.com
http://mothernature.com/ency/herb/

Nellist, CC. "Strategies for Managing Chronic Pelvic Pain." *Ob. Gyn. News* September 15, 1993.

New Zealand National Health Committee. *Guidelines for the Management of Heavy Menstrual Bleeding.* Working Party for Guidelines for the Management of Heavy Menstrual Bleeding, 1998.

Parrott, T. "Using Opioid Analgesics to Manage Chronic Noncancer Pain in Primary Care." *J Am Board Fam Pract* 1999;12(4):293–306. http://www.medscape.com/ABFP/JABFP/1999/v12.n04/fp1204.05.parr/fp1204.05.parr-01.html

Stovall, TG, Ling, FW, Crawford, DA. "Hysterectomy for Chronic Pelvic Pain of Presumed Uterine Etiology." *Obstet Gynec* 1990;75(4):676–679.

Uthman, E. *Understanding Anemia.* Jackson, MS: University Press of Mississippi, 1998.

Wright, JV, Morgenthaler, J (Contributor). *Natural Hormone Replacement for Women Over 45.* Petaluma, CA: Smart Publications, 1997.

Chapter 6 Treat the Fibroids

Myomectomy

"ACOG Technical Bulletin: An Educational Aid to Obstetrician-Gynecologists." *Uterine Leiomyomata.* 1994;192:863–870.

Aziz, A, Petrucco, O, Makinoda, S, Wikholm, G, Svendsen, P, et al. "Transarterial Embolization of the Uterine Arteries: Patient Reactions and Effects on Uterine Vasculature." *Acta Obstet et Gynecologica Scandinavica* 1998;77(3):334–40.

Buttram, V, Reiter, R. "Uterine Leiomyomata: Etiology, Symptomatology, and Management." *Fertility and Sterility* 1981;36(4):433–445.

Dubuisson, JB, Fauconnier, A, Chapron, C, et al. *"Second Look after Laparoscopic Myomectomy."* *Human Reproduction* 1998;13(8):2102–2106.

Greenwood, C, Glickman, M, Schwartz, P, et al. "Obstetric and Nonmalignant Gynecologic Bleeding: Treatment with Angiographic Embolization." *Radiology* 1987;164:155–159.

Hutchins, F. "Abdominal Myomectomy as a Treatment for Symptomatic Uterine Fibroids." *Obstetrics and Gynecology Clinics of North America* 1995;22(4):781–789.

Iverson, R, Chelmow, D, Strohbehn, K, Waldman, L, Evantash, E. "Relative Morbidity of Abdominal Hysterectomy and Myomectomy for Management of Uterine Leiomyomas." *Obstet Gynec* 1996;88(3):415–419.

LaMorte, A, Lalwani, S, Diamond, M. *"Morbidity Associated with Abdominal Myomectomy."* *Obstet Gynec* 1993;82(6).

National Heart, Lung, and Blood Institute (NHLBI). *Transfusion Alert: Use of Autologous Blood.* National Heart, Lung, and Blood Institute Expert Panel on the Use of Autologous Blood, 1995.

Scialli, A. "Alternatives to Hysterectomy for Benign Conditions." *International Journal of Fertility and Women's Medicine* 1998;43 (4):186–91.

Stringer, N, Walker, J, Meyer, P. "Comparison of 49 Laparoscopic Myomectomies with 49 Open Myomectomies." *Journal of the American Association of Gynecologic Laparoscopists* 1997;4(4):457–464.

Sutton, C. "Treatment of Large Uterine Fibroids." *British Journal of Obstetrics and Gynaecology* 1996;103(6):494–6.

Vercellini, P, Maddalena, S, De Giorgi, O, Aimi, G, Crosignani, P. "Abdominal Myomectomy for Infertility: A Comprehensive Review." *Human Reproduction* 1998;13(4):873–879.

Wilcox, L, Lepine, L, Kieke, B. "Comparisons of Hysterectomy or Myomectomy for Uterine Leibomyoma among U.S. Women." *Ahsr and Fhsr Annual Meeting Abstract Book* 1995;1(2):119.

Wilms, G, et al. "Transcatheter Arterial Embolization in the Management of Gynaecological Bleeding." *J Belge Radiol* 1990;73(1):21–5.

Yamashita, Y, Harada, M, Yamamoto, H, et al. "Transcatheter Arterial Embolization of Obstetric and Gynecologic Bleeding: Efficacy and Clinical Outcome." *Br J Radiol* 1994;67:530–534.

Myolysis

Goldfarb, HA. *Does Combining Myoma Coagulation with Endometrial Ablation Reduce Subsequent Surgery?* Montclair Reproductive Center, 1998.

Goldfarb, HA. "Nd:YAG Laser Laparoscopic Coagulation of Symptomatic Myomas." *J Repro Med* 1992;37(7):636–638.

Goldfarb, HA. "Removing Uterine Fibroids Laparoscopically." *Contemporary OB/GYN* 1994;39(2):1–9.

Goldfarb, Herbert. Personal communication.

Hutchins, Francis. Personal communication.

Lyons, Thomas. Personal communication.

Parker, William H. Personal communication.

Phillips, DR, Milim, SJ, Nathanson, JG, Haskelkorn, JS. "Experience with Laparoscopic Leiomyoma Coagulation and Concomitant Operative Hysteroscopy." *J Am Assoc Gynecol Laparosc* 1997;4(4):425–433.

Uterine Artery Embolization (UAE or Uterine Fibroid Embolization—UFE)

Abbara, S, Spies, J, Scialli, A, Jha, R, Lage, J, et al. "Transcervical Expulsion of a Fibroid as a Result of Uterine Artery Embolization of Leiomyomata." *JVIR* 1999;10(4):409–411.

Barr, JD, Lemley, TJ, Petrochko, CN. "Polyvinyl Alcohol Foam Particle Sizes and Concentrations Injectable Through Microcatheters." *JVIR* 1998;9(1):113–118.

Bergman, RA, Afifi, AK, Miyauchi, R. *Anastomoses Between Utero-Ovarian Arteries, Variations. Illustrated Encyclopedia of Human Anatomic Variation: Part II:* "Cardiovascular System." Virtual Hospital International. http://www.vh.org/Providers/Textbooks/AnatomicVariants/Cardiovascular/Images0400/0475.html

Berkowitz, R, Hutchins, F, Worthington-Kirsch, R. "Vaginal Expulsion of Submucosal Fibroids After Uterine Artery Embolization: A Report of Three Cases." *Journal of Reproductive Medicine* 1999;44(4):373–6.

Bradley, E, Reidy, J, Forman, R, Jarosz, J, Braude, P. "Transcatheter Uterine Artery Embolisation to Treat Large Uterine Fibroids." *British Journal of Obstetrics and Gynaecology* 1998;105:235–40.

Broder, MS, Harris, K, Morton, SC, Sherbourne, C, Brook, RH. *Uterine Artery Embolization: A Systematic Review of the Literature and Proposal for Research.* Rand Corporation, 1999.

Broder, MS, Landow, WJ, Goodwin, SC, et al. *"An Agenda for Research into Uterine Artery Embolization: Results of an Expert Panel Conference."* JVIR 2000;11(4):509–515.

Burchell, R. "Physiology of Internal Iliac Artery Ligation." *J. Obstet Gynec* 1968;75:642–651.

Chrisman, HB, Saker, MB, Ryu, RK, Nemcek, AA, et al. "The Impact of Uterine Fibroid Embolization (UFE) on Resumption of Menses and Ovarian Function." At: SCVIR Annual Scientific Meeting, March 2000; San Diego, CA.

Ellis, P, Kelly, I, Fogarty, P. "The Use of Transcatheter Embolisation to Treat Uterine Fibroids." *Ulster Medical Journal* 1998;67(2):139–41.

Goodwin, SC, Chen, G. "Uterine Artery Embolization for Uterine Fibroids." *Contemporary Reviews Obstet & Gynec* 1998.

Goodwin, S, et al. "Uterine Artery Embolization for Uterine Fibroids: Results of a Pilot Study." At: SCVIR Annual Scientific Meeting; March 1997; Washington DC.

Goodwin, S, Lee, M, McLucas, B, Vedantham, S, Fomo, A, Perella, R. "Uterine Artery Embolization for Uterine Fibroids." At: SCVIR Annual Scientific Meeting; March 1998; San Francisco, CA.

Goodwin, S, McLucas, B, Lee, M, Chen, G, Perrella, R, et al. "Uterine Artery Embolization for the Treatment of Uterine Leiomyomata Midterm Results." *JVIR* 1999;10(9):1159–1165.

Goodwin, S, Vedantham, S, McLucas, B, Fomo, A, Perrelia, R. "Preliminary Experience with Uterine Fibroid Embolization for Uterine Fibroids." *JVIR* 1997;8:517–26.

Goodwin, SC, Bonilla, SM, Reed, R, DeCherney, A, Hutchins, F, McCann, L, McLucas, B, Spies, J, Worthington-Kirsch, R, Sacks, D. *Preliminary: Reporting Standards for Uterine Fibroid Embolization,* 2000.

Goodwin, SC, Lai, AC. "Uterine Fibroid Embolization Technique." At: SCVIR Annual Scientific Meeting; March 2000; San Diego, CA.

Goodwin, SC, Landow, WJ, Matalon, TA, et al. "Opportunity and Responsibility: SCVIR's Role with Uterine Artery Embolization." Editorial. *JVIR* 2000;11(4):409–410.

Green, ANH, Walker, WJ. "An Analysis of Results, Complications and Reasons for Failure Following Bilaterial Uterine Embolization." Royal Surrey County Hospital. Personal Communication.

Gupta A, Shlansky-Goldberg, RD, Tureck, RW, Cobb, PG, Soulen, MC, Baum, RA, et al. "Post-Procedural Pain Following Uterine Artery Embolization Does not Correlate with Outcome." At: SCVIR Annual Scientific Meeting; March 2000; San Diego, CA.

Hutchins, F, Worthington-Kirsch, R, Berkowitz, R. "Selective Uterine Artery Embolization as Primary Treatment for Symptomatic Leiomyomata Uteri." *J Amer Assoc Gynecol Laparosc* 1999;6(3):279–84.

Katsumori, T, Nakajima, K, Hanada, Y. "MR Imaging of a Uterine Myoma after Embolization." *American Journal of Roentgenology* 1999;172(1):248–9.

Katz, R, Mitty, H, Stancato-Pasik, A, Cooper, J, Ahn, J. "Comparison of Uterine Artery Embolization for Fibroids Using Gelatin Sponge Pledgets and Polyvinyl Alcohol." At: SCVIR Annual Scientific Meeting; March 1998; San Francisco, CA.

Kuhn, R, Mitchell, P. "Embolic Occlusion of the Blood Supply to Uterine Myomas: Report of 2 Cases." *Australian & New Zealand Journal of Obstetrics & Gynaecology* 1999;39:1:120–2.

Lai, AC, Goodwin, SC, Bonilla, SM, Lai, AP, Yegul, T, Vott, S, DeLeon, M. "Sexual Dysfunction after Uterine Artery Embolization." *JVIR* 2000;11(6):755–758.

Ledreff, Pelage J, Dahan, H, Kardache, M, Jacob, D, Rymer, R. "Arterial Embolization for Uterine Leiomyomata: Nfid-Term Results with Focus on Bleeding." At: RSNA Scientific Assembly and Annual Meeting; November 1998; Chicago, IL.

Lipman, JC. "Uterine Artery Embolization for the Treatment of Symptomatic Uterine Fibroids: A Review." *Applied Radiology* 2000;7:15–20.

Nikolic, B, Spies, JB, Abbara, S, et al. "Ovarian Artery Supply of Uterine Fibroids as a Cause of Treatment Failure after Uterine Artery Embolization: A Case Report." JVIR 1999; 10 (9): 1167–1170.

Nikolic, B, Spies, JB, Lundsten, MJ, et al."Patient Radiation Dose Associated with Uterine Artery Embolization." *Radiology* 2000;214(1):121–125.

Pelage, JP, Soyer, P, Repiquet, D, et al. "Secondary Postpartum Hemorrhage: Treatment with Selective Arterial Embolization." *Radiology* 1999;212(2):385–389.

Poppe, W, Van Assche, FA, Wilms, G, Favril, A, Baert, A. "Pregnancy after Transcatheter Embolization of a Uterine Arteriovenous Malformation." *Am J Obstet Gynecol* 1987;156(5):1179–1180.

Pron, G, Common, A, Sniderman, K. "Radiological Embolization of Uterine Arteries of Symptomatic Fibroids: Preliminary Findings of a Canadian Multicenter Trial." At: SCVIR Annual Scientific Meeting; March 1999; Orlando, FL.

Ravina, JH, Vigneron, NC, Aymard, A, et al. *Pregnancy after embolization of uterine myoma: report of 12 cases.* Fertility and Sterility 2000;73(6):1241–1243.

Ravina, J, et al. "Arterial Embolization: A New Treatment of Menorrhagia in Uterine Fibroma." *La Presse Medicale.* 1995; 24(37):1754.

Ravina, J, Aymard, A, Bouret, J, Ciraru-Vigneron, N, Houdart, E, et al. "Particulate Arterial Embolization: A New Treatment for Uterine Leiomyomata-Related Hemorrhage." La Presse Medicale 1998;27:299–303.

Ravina, J, Bouret, J, et al. *Application of Particulate Arterial Embolization in the Treatment of Uterine Fibromyomata.* *Bulletin, the French National Academy of Medicine* 1997;181(2).

Ravina, J, Bouret, J, Ciraru-Vigneron, N, Repiquet, D, Herbreteau, D, et al. "Recourse to Particulate Arterial Embolization in the Treatment of Some Uterine Leiomyoma." *Bulletin de L'academie Nationale Medicine* 1997;181(2):233–43.

Ravina, J, Bouret, J, Fried, D, et al. "Value of Preoperative Embolization of Uterine Fibroma: Report of a Multicenter Series of 31 Cases." *Contraception, Fertilitie, Sexualitie* 1995;23:45–49.

Ravina, J, Ciraru-Vigneron, N, Aymard, A, Ledreff, O, Herbreteau, D, Merland, J. "Arterial Embolization of Uterine Myomata: Results of 184 Cases." SMIT, September 1998; London, England.

Ravina, J, Herbreteau, D, Ciraru-Vigneron, N, Bouret, J, Houdart, E, et al. "Arterial Embolisation to Treat Uterine Myomata." *Lancet* 1995; 346:671–2.

Ravina, J, Merland, J, Herbreteau, D, Houdart, E, Bouret, J, et al. "Preoperative Embolization of Uterine Fibroma. Preliminary Results (10 Cases)." *La Presse Medicale* 1994; 23(33):1540.

Reidy, J, Bradley, E. "Uterine Artery Embolization for Fibroid Disease." *Cardiovascular and Interventional Radiology* 1998;21(5):357–60.

Roth, AR, Spies, JB, Walsh, EL, Wood, B, Gomez-Jorge, J. "Pain after Uterine Fibroid Embolization: Prediction of Severity and Relevance to Outcome." At: SCVIR Annual Scientific Meeting; March 2000; San Diego, CA.

Schifano, MJ, Hoshaw, NJ, Boushka, WM, et al. "Uterine Artery Embolization in a Hemorrhaging Postoperative Myomectomy Patient." Editorial. *Obstet Gynecol Surv* 1999;54(1):1–4.

SCVIR. "Uterine Fibroid Embolization. New Advances in Women's Health Care, A National Meeting Conference Program." October 22–23, 1999.

Siskin, GP, Stainken, BF, Dowling, K, Meo, P, Ahn, J, Dolen, E. "Outpatient Uterine Artery Embolization for Symptomatic Uterine Fibroids: Experience in 49 Patients." *JVIR* 2000;11(3):305–311.

Smith, SJ. "Uterine Fibroid Embolization." *Am Fam Physician* 2000, 61(12):3601–3607.

Spies, J, Barth, K, Scialli, A, Jha, R, Ascher, S, Lossef, S. "Uterine Artery Embolization for Uterine Fibroids: Initial Experience and Short-term Outcome." At: RSNA Scientific Assembly and Annual Meeting; November, 1998; Chicago, IL.

Spies, J, Jha, R, Ascher, S, Barth, K, Losef, S, Walsh, S. "Uterine Artery Embolization of Symptomatic Fibroids: Short-term Results." *JVIR*. At: SCVIR Annual Scientific Meeting; March 1999; Orlando, FL.

Spies, J, Scialli, AR, JHA, R, Imaoka, I, Ascher, SM, Fraga, VM, Barth, KH. "Initial Results from Uterine Fibroid Embolization for Symptomatic Leiomyomata." *JVIR* 1999;10(9):1149–1157.

Spies, J, Warren, EH, Mathias, SD, Wash, SM, Roth, AR, Pentecost, MJ. "Uterine Fibroid Embolization: Measurement of Health-Related Quality of Life before and after Therapy." *JVIR* 1999;10(10):1293–1303.

Stancato-Pasik, A, Mitty, H, Katz, R, Braffman, B, Shapairo, R, Brodman, M. "Embolization of Uterine Myomas: Sonographic Assessment and Clinical Follow-Up." At: SCVIR Annual Scientific Meeting; March 1998; San Francisco, CA.

Stancato-Pasik, A, Mitty, HA, Richard, HM, III, Eshkar, N. "Obstetric Embolotherapy: Effect on Menses and Pregnancy." *Radiology* 1997;204(3): 791–793.

Sterling, KM, Cooper, JM. "Patient Evaluation and Preparation." Symposium on Gynecologic Intervention. At: SCVIR Annual Scientific Meeting; March 2000; San Diego, CA.

Vashist, A, Studd, J, Carey, A, Burn, P. "Fatal Septicemia after Fibroid Embolization." *Lancet* 1999;354:307–308.

Vedantham, S, Goodwin, S, McLucas, B, Mohr, G. "Uterine Artery Embolization: An Underused Method of Controlling Pelvic Hemorrhage." *American Journal of Obstetrics and Gynecology* 1997; 176(4):938–948.

Vedantham, S, Goodwin, SC, McLucas, B, et al. "Uterine Artery Embolization for Fibroids: Considerations in Patient Selection and Clinical Follow-Up." *Medscape Womens Health* 1999;4(5):2.

Walker, W. "Bilateral Uterine Artery Embolization for Fibroids," in *Menorrhagia,* Chapter 16. Sheth, S, Sutton, S, eds. Oxford, England: Isis Medical Media, June 1999.

Worthington-Kirsch, R, Popky, G, Hutchins, F. "Uterine Arterial Embolization for the Management of Leiomyomas: Quality-of-life Assessment and Clinical Response." *Radiology.* 1998; 208:625–9.

Worthington-Kirsch, R. "Flow Redistribution During Uterine Artery Embolization for the Management of Symptomatic Fibroids." *JVIR* 1999; 10(2):237–8.

Hysterectomy
Alexander, DA, Naji, AA, Pinion, SB, et al. "Randomised Trial Comparing Hysterectomy with Endometrial Ablation for Dysfunctional Uterine Bleeding: Psychiatric and Psychosocial Aspects." *BMJ* 1996; 312:280–284.

American College of Obstetricians & Gynecologists. *Hysterectomy.* Patient Education Pamphlet, 1995.

Amirikia, H, Evans, TN. "Ten-Year Review of Hysterectomies: Trends, Indications, and Risks." *Am J Obstet Gynecol* 1979;134:431–437.

Angle, HS, Cohen, SM, Hidlebaugh, D. "The Initial Worcester Experience with Laparoscopic Hysterectomy." *J Am Assoc Gynecol Laparosc* 1995(2):155–161.

Apoola, A, Hefni, MA. "Hysterectomy for Moderately Enlarged Uterus: Abdominal Versus Vaginal Hysterectomy." *J Obstet Gynec* 1998; 18(4):375–376.

Averette, HE, Hoskins, W, Nyuyen, HN, et al. "National Survey of Ovarian Carcinoma. A Patient Care Evaluation Study of the American College of Surgeons, Cancer Supplement." February 13, 1993;71(4):1629–1638.

Bateman, BG, Kolp, LA, Hoeger, K. "Complications of Laparoscopy—Operative and Diagnostic." *Fertil Steril* 1996;66:30–35.

Benjamin, BC. *Hysterectomy: A Primer.* Haverford 5/16/1996.http://www.students.haverford.edu/wmbweb/topics/hysterectomy.html

Bernstein, S, Fiske, M, McGlynn, E, Gifford, D. *Hysterectomy: A review of the Literature on Indications, Effectiveness, and Risks.* Santa Monica, CA: RAND, 1997. Publication MR-592/2-ACHPR.

Boike, GM, Elfstrand, EP, DelPriore, G, Schumock, D, Holley, HS, Lurain, JR. "Laparoscopically Assisted Vaginal Hysterectomies in a University Hospital: Report of 82 Cases and Comparison with Abdominal and Vaginal Hysterectomy." *Am J Obstet Gynecol* 1993;168:1690–1701.

Bolger, BS, Lopes, T, Monaghan, JM. "Laparoscopically Assisted Vaginal Hysterectomy: A Report of the First 300 Completed Procedures." *Gynaecol Endosc* 1997;6:77–81.

Bronitsky, C, Payne, RJ, Stuckey, S, Wilkins, D. "A Comparison of Laparoscopically Assisted Vaginal Hysterectomy vs Traditional Totalabdominal and Vaginal Hysterectomies." *J Gynecol Surg* 1993;219:224.

Brown, R, Erian, J. "Cervical Conservation: The Future of Hysterectomy?" *Gynaecol Endosc* 1996;5:211–216.

Canis, M, Mage, G, Chapron, C, Wattiez, A, Pouly, JL, Bruhat, MA. "Laparoscopic Hysterectomy: A Preliminary Study." *Surg Endosc* 1993;7:42–45.

Carlson, KJ, Miller, BA, Fowler, FJ, Jr. "The Maine Women's Health Study, I: Outcomes of Hysterectomy." *Obstet Gynecol* 1994; 83:556–565.

Chakravarti, S, Collins, WP, Newton, JR, Oram, DH, Studd, J. "Endocrine Changes and Symptomology after Oophorectomy in Premenopausal Women." *Br J Obstet Gynaecol* 1977; 84:769–775.

Chapron, C, Dubuisson, J-B, Ansquer, Y. "Hysterectomy for Patients without Previous Vaginal Delivery: Results and Modalities of Laparoscopic Surgery." *Hum Reprod* 1996;11:2122–2126.

Chapron, C, Dubuisson, J-B, Aubert, V, Morice, P, Garnier, P, Aubriot, F-X, Foulot, H. "Total Laparoscopic Hysterectomy: Preliminary Results." *Hum Reprod* 1994;9:2084–2089.

Chapron, C, Pierre, F, Harchaoui, Y, Lacroix, S, Béguin, S, Querleu, D, Lansac, J, Dubuisson, J-B. "Gastrointestinal Injuries During Gynaecological Laparoscopy." *Hum Reprod* 1999;14:333–337.

Chapron, C, Querleu, D, Bruhat, M-A, Madelenat, P, Fernandez, H, Pierre, F, Dubuisson, J-B. "Surgical Complications of Diagnostic and Operative Gynaecological Laparoscopy: A Series of 29,966 Cases." *Hum Reprod* 1998;13:867–872.

Chapron, CM, Pierre, F, Lacroix, S, Querleu, D, Lansac, J, Dubuisson, J-B. "Major Vascular Injuries During Gynecologic Laparoscopy." *J Am Coll Surg* 1997a;185:461–465.

Coppen, A, Bishop, M, Beard, RJ, Barnard, GJR, Collins, WP. "Hysterectomy, Hormones, and Behavior." *Lancet* 1981; 1:126–128.

Cosson, M, Rajabally, R, Querleu, D, Crepin, G. "Hysterectomy: Indications, Surgical Routes, Cases for Adnexal or Cervical Conservation." *Eur J Obstet Gynecol Reprod Biol* 1995;80:5–15.

Davies, A, Vizza, E, Bournas, N, O'Connor, H, Magos, A. "How to Increase the Proportion of Hysterectomies Performed Vaginally." *Am J Obstet Gynecol* 1998;179:1008–1012.

Dicker, RG, Greenspan, JR, Strauss, LT, Cowart, MR, Scally, MJ, Peterson, HB, DeStefano, F, Rubin, GL, Ory, HW. "Complications of Abdominal and Vaginal Hysterectomy among Women of Reproductive Age in the United States." *Am J Obstet Gynecol* 1982;144:841–848.

Donnez, J, Nisolle, M, Smets, M, Polet, R, Bassil, S. "Laparoscopic Supracervical (Subtotal) Hysterectomy: A First Series of 500 Cases." *Gynaecol Endosc* 1997;6:73–76.

Dorsey, JH, Steinberg, EP, Holtz, PM. "Clinical Indications for Hysterectomy Route: Patient Characteristics or Physician Preference?" *Am J Obstet Gynecol* 1995;173:1452–1460.

Easterday, CL, Grimes, DA, Riggs, JA. "Hysterectomy in the United States." *Obstet Gynecol* 1983;62:203–212.

Falcone, T, Paraiso, MFR, Mascha, E. *"Prospective Randomized Clinical Trial of Laparoscopically Assisted Vaginal Hysterectomy Versus Total Abdominal Hysterectomy."* *Am J Obstet Gynecol* 1999;180:955–962.

Garry, R. "Complications of Laparoscopic Entry." *Gynaecol Endosc* 1997;6:319–329.

Garry, R. "Towards Evidence-Based Hysterectomy." *Gynaecol Endosc* 1998;7:225–233.

Garry, R, Phillips, G. "How Safe is the Laparoscopic Approach to Hysterectomy?" *Gynaecol Endosc* 1995;4:77–79.

Gates, EA. "New Surgical Procedures: Can Our Patients Benefit While We Learn?" *Am J Obstet Gynecol* 1997;176:1293–1299.

Gath, D, Cooper, P, Day, A. "Hysterectomy and Psychiatric Disorder, I: Levels of Psychiatric Morbidity Before and After Hysterectomy." *Br J Psychiatry* 1982; 140:335–350.

Giesler, CF. "The Texas Approach to Total Laparoscopic Hysterectomy." http://www.reproductivecenter.com/texas.html

Gitsch, G, Berger, E, Tatra, G. "Trends in Thirty Years of Vaginal Hysterectomy." *Surg Gynecol Obstet* 1991;172:207–210.

Goodwin, JS, Hunt, WC, Key, CCR, Samet, JM. "Changes in Surgical Treatments: The Example of Hysterectomy Versus Conization for Cervical Carcinoma in Situ." *J Clin Epidemiol* 1990;43(9)977–982.

Härkki-Sirén, P. "Laparoscopic Hysterectomy: Outcome and Complications in Finland." Department of Obstetrics and Gynecology. Helsinki University Central Hospital, University of Helsinki, Finland. Academic dissertation presented 11/5/1999.

Harris, MB, Olive, DL. "Changing Hysterectomy Patterns after Introduction of Laparoscopically Assisted Vaginal Hysterectomy." *Am J Obstet Gynecol* 1994;171:340–344.

Harris, WJ, Daniell, JF. "Early Complications of Laparoscopic Hysterectomy." *Obstet Gynecol Surv* 1996;51:559–567.

Hasson, HM. "Cervical Removal at Hysterectomy for Benign Disease: Risks and Benefits." *J Reprod Med.* 1993;38:781–790.

Hill, V, Overton, C, Hargreaves, J, Maresh, MJA. "Hysterectomy in the Treatment of Dysfunctional Uterine Bleeding." *Br J Obstet Gynaecol* 1998b;105(S17):60.

Ikhena, S, Oni, M, Naftalin, NJ, Konje, JC. "The Effect of the Learning Curve on the Duration and Peri-Operative Complications of Laparoscopically Assisted Vaginal Hysterectomy." *Acta Obstet Gynecol Scand* 1999;78:632–635.

Jansen FW, Kapiteyn, K, Trimbox-Kemper, T, Hermans, J, Trimbos, JB. "Complications of Laparoscopy: A Prospective Multicentre Observational Study." *Br J Obstet Gynaecol* 1997;104:595–600.

Johns, DA, Carrera, B, Jones, J, DeLeon, F, Vincent, R., Safely, C. "The Medical and Economic Impact of Laparoscopically Assisted Vaginal Hysterectomy in a Large, Metropolitan, Not-for-Profit Hospital." *Am J Obstet Gynecol* 1995;172:1709–1719.

Kadar, N, Pelosi, MA. "Laparoscopically Assisted Hysterectomy in Women Weighing 200 lb or More." *Gynaecol Endosc* 1994;5:159–162.

Kauko, M. "New Techniques Using the Ultrasonic Scalpel in Laparoscopic Hysterectomy." *Curr Opin Obstet Gynecol* 1998;10:303–305.

Kore, S, Sah, A, Hegde, A, Srikrishna, S, Ambiye, V. "Bisection, Myomectomy and Coring in Vaginal Hysterectomy of Large Uterus." *Bombay Hospital Journal* 1999;41(4).

Kramer, MG, Reiter, RC. "Hysterectomy: Indications, Alternatives and Predictors." *American Family Physician* 1997; 55(3):827–835.

Kudo, R, Yamauchi, O, Okazaki, T, Sagae, S, Ito, E, Hashimoto, M. "Vaginal Hysterectomy without Ligation of the Ligaments of the Cervix Uteri." *Surg Gynecol Obstet* 1990;170:299–305.

Lambden, MP, Bellamy, G, Ogburn-Russell, L, et al. "Women's Sense of Well-Being before and after Hysterectomy." *J Obstet Gynecol Neonatal Nursing* 1997; 26:540–548.

Lécuru, F, Darles, C, Robin, F, Huss, M, Ruscillo, M, Taurelle, R. "Morbidity of Routine Gynaecological Laparoscopy: Report of a Series of 283 Procedures." *Gynaecol Endosc* 1996;5:79–82.

Lilford, RJ. "Hysterectomy: Will It Pay the Bills in 2007?" *BMJ* 1997;314(7075):160–162.

Liu, CY, Reich, H. "Complications of Total Laparoscopic Hysterectomy in 518 Cases." *Gynaecol Endosc* 1994;3:203–208.

Lyons, TL. "Laparoscopic Supracervical Hysterectomy." *Baill Clin Obstet Gynecol* 1997;11:167–180.

Magos, A, Bournas, N, Sinha, R, Richardson, RE, O'Connor, H. "Vaginal Hysterectomy for the Large Uterus." *Br J Obstet Gynaecol* 1996;103:246–251.

Marana, R, Busacca, M, Zupi, E, Garcea, N, Paparella, P, Catalano, GF. "Laparoscopically Assisted Vaginal Hysterectomy Versus Total Abdominal Hysterectomy: A Prospective, Randomized, Multicenter Study." *Am J Obstet Gynecol* 1999;180:270–275.

Meikle, SF, Nugent, EW, Orleans, M. "Complications and Recovery from Laparoscopy-Assisted Vaginal Hysterectomy with Abdominal and Vaginal Hysterectomy." *Obstet Gynecol* 1997;89:304–311.

Mencaglia, L, Van Herendael, B, Tantini, C, Stampini, A. "Laparoscopic-Assisted Vaginal Hysterectomy: Evaluation of Benefits of Laparoscopic Hysterectomy." *Gynaecol Endosc* 1994;3:209–211.

Mettler, L, Lutzewitch, N, Dewitz, T, Remmert, K, Semm, K. "From Laparotomy to Pelviscopic Intrafascial Hysterectomy." *Gynaecol Endosc* 1996;5:203–209.

Munro, MG, Deprest, J. "Laparoscopic Hysterectomy: Does It Work?: A Bicontinental Review of the Literature and Clinical Commentary." *Clin Obstet Gynecol* 1995;2:401–425.

Nawaz, H, Katz, D. "Perimenopausal and Postmenopausal Hormone Replacement Therapy." *Am J Prev Med* 1999; 17(3):250–254.

Olsson, J-H, Ellström, M, Hahlin, M. "A Randomised Trial Comparing Laparoscopic and Abdominal Hysterectomy." *Br J Obstet Gynaecol* 1996;103:345–350.

Optimed Medical Systems. "Hysterectomy." In: Hysterectomy Protocols, Version 6.1 (software), 1997.

Ou, C-S, Beadle, E, Preshus, J, Smith, M. "A Multicenter Review of 839 Laparoscopic-Assisted Vaginal Hysterectomies." *J Am Assoc Gynecol Laparosc* 1994;1:417–422.

Padial, JG, Sotolongo, J, Casey, MJ, Johnson, C, Osborne, NG. "Laparoscopy-Assisted Vaginal Hysterectomy: Report of Seventy-Five Consecutive Cases." *J Gynecol Surg* 1992;8:81–85.

Phipps, JH, John, M, Hassamaien, M, Saced, M. "Laparoscopic and Laparoscopically Assisted Vaginal Hysterectomy—A Series of 114 Cases." *Gynaecol Endosc* 1993;2:7–12.

Phipps, JH, Nayak, JS. "Comparison of Laparoscopically Assisted Vaginal Hysterectomy and Bilateral Salpingo-Ophorectomy with Conventional Abdominal Hysterectomy and Bilateral Salpingo-Ophorectomy." *Br J Obstet Gynaecol* 1993;100:698–700.

Raju, KS, Auld, BJ. "A Randomized Prospective Study of Laparoscopic Vaginal Hysterectomy Versus Abdominal Hysterectomy Each with Bilateral Salpingo-Oophorectomy." *Br J Obstet Gynaecol* 1994;101:1068–1071.

Reich, H, DeCaprio, J, McGlynn, F. "Laparoscopic Hysterectomy." *J Gynecol Surg* 1989;5:213–216.

Reich, H, McGlynn, F, Sekel, L. "Total Laparoscopic Hysterectomy." *Gynaecol Laparosc* 1993;2:59–63.

Richards, DH. "A Post-Hysterectomy Syndrome." *Lancet* 1974;2:983–985.

Richardson, RE, Bournas, N, Magos, AL. "Is Laparoscopic Hysterectomy a Waste of Time?" *Lancet* 1995;345:36–41.

Rosen, DMB, Cario, GM, Carlton, MA, Lam, AM. "Return to Work Following Laparoscopic Hysterectomy." *Gynaecol Endosc* 1997;6:261–264.

Rosen, DMB, Cario, GM, Carlton, MA, Lam, AM, Chapman, M. "An Assessment of the Learning Curve for Laparoscopic and Total Laparoscopic Hysterectomy." *Gynaecol Endosc* 1998;7:289–293.

Roushdy, M. "Vaginally Assisted Laparoscopic Hysterectomy: A Technique Suited for Large Uteri." *Gynaecol Endosc* 1997;6:95–97.

Roushdy, M, Farag, O, Mosaad, M, Zayed, M. "Pain after Hysterectomy: A Comparison Between Four Currently Available Procedures." *Gynaecol Endosc* 1997;6:99–103.

Rowe, M, Kanouse, D, Mittman, B, Bernstein, S. "Quality of Life Among Women Undergoing Hysterectomies." *Journal of Obstetrics and Gynecology* 1999;93(6):915–920.

Schofield, MJ, Bennett, A, Redman, S, Walters, WAW, Sanson-Fisher, RW. "Self-Reported Long-Term Outcomes of Hysterectomy." *Br J Obstet Gynaecol* 1991; 98:1129–1136.

Scott, JR, Sharp, HT, Dodson, MK, Norton, PA, Warner, HR. "Subtotal Hysterectomy in Modern Gynecology: A Decision Analysis." *Am J Obstet Gynecol* 1997;176:1186–1192.

Sills, ES, Saini, J, Steiner, CA, McGee, III, M, Gretz, III, HF. "Abdominal Hysterectomy Practice Patterns in the United States." *Intl J of Gyn & Obstet* 1998; 63:277–283.

Society of Pelvic Reconstructive Surgeons—Medical Specialty Society. *Guideline for Determining the Route and Method of Hysterectomy for Benign Conditions,* 1999.

Tsaltas, J, Magnus, A, Mamers, PM, Lawrence, AS, Lolatgis, N, Healy, D. "Laparoscopic and Abdominal Hysterectomy: A Cost Comparison." *MJA* 1997;166:205.

Van Den Eeden, SK, Glasser, M, Mathias, SD, Colwell, HH, Pasta, DJ, Kunz, K. "Quality of Life, Health Care Utilization, and Costs Among Women Undergoing Hysterectomy in a Managed-Care Setting." *Am J Obstet Gynecol* 1998;178(1)91–100.

Clinical Trials

Agency for Health Care Policy and Research. *AHCPR: Improving Health Care Quality Through Research and Education.* AHCPR Pub. No. 99-P007, 10/99. http://www.ahcpr.gov/news/profile.htm

CenterWatch. *Background Information on Clinical Research.* Clinical Trials Listing Service™ 10/5/99. http://www.centerwatch.com/backgrnd.htm

ClinicalTrials.gov
National Library of Medicine
http://www.clinicaltrials.gov

National Institutes of Health. *What Is a Clinical Trial?*
http://www.nih.gov/health/

Lupron

Department of Health and Human Services, Office of Inspector General. United States Federal Register: May 1, 1996;61(85):19295–19296. From the Federal Register Online via GPO Access: http://wais.access.gpo.gov

Foreman, Judy. "Treatment Options are Growing for Women With Bleeding Disorders." *The Boston Globe,* March 23, 1998.

Lasalandra, Michael. "Noted Doc Loses License for Falsifying Med Data," *Boston Herald,* June 2, 1998, p. 16.

Lazar, Kay. "Wonder Drug in Men Alleged to Cause Harm in Women." *Boston Herald,* August 22, 23, 24, 1999 (3 part series).

Lupron TAP Pharmaceuticals
http://www.lupron.com

Massachusetts Board of Registration in Medicine, In the Matter of Andrew J. Friedman. Final Decision & Order, No. 97-21-DALA, May 20, 1998. See www.docboard.org under the physician's name for updates.

Mesia, AF, Williams, FS, Yan, Z, Mittal, K. "Aborted Leiomyosarcoma after Treatment with Leuprolide Acetate." *Obstet & Gynec* 1998;92(4, part 2):664–666.

The National Lupron Victims Network.
http://www.lupronvictims.com

Retraction of Friedman, A. J. et al., "Gonadotropin-releasing hormone agonist plus estrogin-progestin 'add-back' therapy for endometriosis-related pelvic pain" in *Fertil Steril* 1996; 65(1):211.

Retraction of Friedman, A. J. et al., "Does low-dose combination oral contraceptive use affect uterine size or menstrual flow in premenopausal women with leiomyomas" in *Obstet Gynecol* 1995; 86(5):728.

Rintala, S, Kujansuu, E, Teisala, K, Rantala, I, Kivinen, S, Tuimala, R. "GnRH Analogues and Uterine Leiomyomas: Effect of Hormone Replacement Therapy on Cell Proliferation." *Gynecol Obstet Invest* 1999;48(4):276–279.

TAP Pharmaceuticals
http://www.tap.com

Mifepristone (RU-486)

"The Abortion Pill's Grim Progress" (editorial). *Mother Jones* 1999: n24v1.

Blumenthal, P, Johnson, J, Stewart, F. "The Approval of Mifepristone (RU-486) in the United States. What's Wrong with This Picture?" *Medscape* 2000:5(4). http://www.medscape.com/Medscape/WomensHealth/journal/2000/v5.n04/wh0726.blum/wh0726.blum-01.html

The Danco Group. Personal communication. (Manufacturer/Distributor.)

Steven H. Eisinger. Personal communication. (Uterine fibroid research.)

Feminist Majority Foundation. http://www.feminist.org

Fraser, L. "The Abortion Pill's Grim Progress." *Mother Jones* Jan/Feb 1999. http://www.mojones.com/mother_jones/JF99/wellbeing1.html

Kettel, LM, Murphy, AA, Morales, AJ, Ulmann, A, Baulieu, EE, Yen, SSC. "Treatment of Endometriosis with the Antiprogesterone Mifepristone (RU486)." *Fertility & Sterility* 1995;65(1):23–28.

Heleen LeRoux. Personal communication. (Uterine fibroid research.)

Murphy, AA, Kettel, LM, Morales, AJ, Roberts, VJ, Parmley, T, Yen, SSC. "Endometrial Effects of Long-Term Low-Dose Administration of RU486." *Fertility & Sterility* 1995;63(4):761–766.

Murphy, AA, Kettel, LM, Morales, AJ, Roberts, VJ, Yen, SSC. "Regression of Uterine Leiomyomata in Response to the Antiprogesterone RU486." *J Clin Endoc and Metab* 1993;76(2):513–517.

Murphy, AA, Morales, AJ, Kettel, LM, Yen, SSC. "Regression of Uterine Leiomyomata to the Antiprogesterone RU486: Dose-Response Effect." *Fertility & Sterility* 1995;64(1):18–190.

Nettleton, S. Payne. Personal communication. (Brain tumor research.)

Eric, A. Schaff. Personal communication. (Uterine fibroid research.)

Talbot, Margaret. "The Little White Bombshell." *New York Times Magazine,* July 11, 1999.

Samuel S. Yen. Personal communication. (Endometriosis research.)

Female Reconstructive Surgery
California Medical Board.
http://www.docboard.org/ca/df/casearch.htm

Coalition for Post Tubal Women
http://www.hormonecheck.com

Department of Health and Human Services, Office of Inspector General. United States Federal Register: September 21, 1999 (v 64, n 182, p. 51128–51132.)
Federal Register Online via GPO Access: http://wais.access.gpo.gov [DOCID:fr21se99-63]

europahealth.com

Cycles newsletter, volume 1 issue 1, September 1999.
Cycles newsletter, volume 1 issue 2, December 1999.
Cycles newsletter, volume 2 issue 1, Spring 2000.

The Federation of State Medical Boards.
http://www.fsmb.org

Hufnagel, VG. Personal communication.

Hufnagel, VG. web pages:
http://www.drhufnagel.com
http://www.nomorehysterectomies.com
http://www.drhufnagel.com/rama1.html
http://www.drhufnagel.com/library.html
http://www.drhufnagel.com/sellingsurgery.html
http://www.drhufnagel.com/nomoremenopausetext.html
http://www.nomoremenopause.com
http://www.hypatiapub.com
http://www.tubal.org

Hufnagel, VG and SK Golant (Contributor). *No More Hysterectomies*. New York: Plume, 1989.

New York Medical Board.
http://www.health.state.ny.us/nysdoh/opmc/news/98/98feb.htm#hufnagel
http://www.health.state.ny.us/nysdoh/commish/98/hufnagel.htm

Legal Records:

Division of Medical Quality, Board of Medical Quality Assurance, Department of Consumer Affairs, State of California v. *V. Georges Hufnagel.* Record D-3613. February 26, 1987.

Division of Medical Quality, Board of Medical Quality Assurance, Department of Consumer Affairs, State of California v. *V. Georges Hufnagel.* Record L-39699. Decision: December 30, 1988. Notice of Non-Adoption of Proposed Decision: March 6, 1989.

Division of Medical Quality, Board of Medical Quality Assurance, Department of Consumer Affairs, State of California, In the Matter of the Accusation Against V. Georges Hufnagel. Decision, No. D-3616, L-39699, August 14, 1989.

V. Georges Hufnagel v. *Division of Medical Quality, Board of Medical Quality Assurance, Department of Consumer Affairs, State of California.* Case No C 730 624. Statement of Decision: July 19, 1996.

V Georges Hufnagel v. *Division of Medical Quality, Board of Medical Quality Assurance, Department of Consumer Affairs, State of California.* Case No C 730 624. Judge Denying Petition for Writ of Mandate: September 3, 1996.

Legal Information Institute
Orders in Pending Cases for May 26, 1998
Section: CERTIORARI DENIED
97-1586 HUFNAGEL, VICKI V. MEDICAL BD. OF CA
http://supct.law.cornell.edu/supct/html/052698.ZOR.html

State of New York, Department of Health. Administrative Review Board (ARB) Determination and Order 98-33. In the Matter of V. Georges Hufnagel. June 29, 1998.

Chapter 7 Related Health Issues

Ahn, C, Lee, WH, Sunwoo, TW, Kho, YS. "Uuterine Arterial Embolization for the Treatment of Symptomatic Adenomyosis of the Uterus." At: SCVIR Annual Scientific Meeting; March 2000; San Diego, CA.

Amais, AG. "Sexual Life After Gynaecological Operations." *BMJ* 1975 2:608–609.

Bachmann, GA. "Psychosexual Aspects of Hysterectomy." *Womens Health Issues* 1990; 1:41–49.

Bickerstaff, H. "The Presurgical Diagnosis of Diffuse Adenomyosis." *European Assoc Gyn & Obstet Newsletter* 1996;2(2). Published summer 1997. http://www.obgyn.net/eago/art04.htm

Carlson, KJ, Miller, BA, Fowler, FJ. "The Maine Women's Health Study, II: Outcomes of Nonsurgical Management of Leiomyomas, Abnormal Bleeding, and Chronic Pelvic Pain." *Obstet Gynecol* 1994; 83:566–572.

Center for Uterine Fibroids. *"Fibroid-Like Conditions: Adenomyosis."* OBGYN.net Publications 2000. http://www.obgn.net/AH/articles/Adenomyosis.htm

Craig, GA, Jackson, P. "Sexual Life after Vaginal Hysterectomy." *BMJ* 1975 3:97.

Darling, CA, McKoy-Smith, YM. "Understanding Hysterectomies: Sexual Satisfaction and Quality of Life." *The Journal of Sex Research* 1993:30(4):324–335.

Davis, MA. "Sexuality and Sexual Dysfunction." *Journal of Psychology* November 1998.

Dennerstein, L, Wood, C, Burrows, GD. "Sexual Response Following Hysterectomy and Oopherectomy." *Obstet Gynecol* 1977 49:92–96.

Drife, J. "Conserving the Cervix at Hysterectomy." Commentaries. *Br J Obstet Gynaecol* 1994;101:563–564.

Edwards, JG, Anderson, I. "Systematic Review and Guide to Selection of Selective Serotonin Reuptake Inhibitors." *Drugs* 1999;57(4):507–533.

Ewert, B, Slangen, T, van Herendael, B. "Sexuality after Laparoscopic-Assisted Vaginal Hysterectomy." *J Am Assoc Gynecol Laparosc* 1995;3:27–32.

Francis, WJA, Jeffcoate, TNA. "Dyspareunia Following Vaginal Operations." *J Obstet Gynaecol Br Commonw* 1961; 68:1–10.

Glass, C, Soni, B. "Sexual Problems of Disabled Patients." *BMJ* 1999;318 (7182):518–511.

Goodman, MT, Wilkens, LR, Hankin, JH, Lyu, LC, Wu, AH, Kolonel, LN. "Association of Soy and Fiber Consumption with the Risk of Endometrial Cancer." *American Journal of Epidemiology* 1997;146(4):294–306.

Helström, L, Weiner, E, Sörbom, D, Bäckström, T. "Predictive Value of Psychiatric History, Genital Pain and Menstrual Symptoms for Sexuality after Hysterectomy." *Acta Obstet Gynecol Scand* 1994;73:575–580.

Helström, L, Lundberg, PO, Sörbom, D, Bäckström, T. "Sexuality after Hysterectomy: A Factor Analysis of Women's Sexual Lives before and after Subtotal Hysterectomy." *Obstet Gynecol* 1993 81:357–362.

Hitt, Jack. "The Second Sexual Revolution." *NY Times Magazine* February 20, 2000.

Huffman, W. "The Effect of Gynecologic Surgery on Sexual Reactions." *Am J Obstet Gynecol.* 1950;59:915–917.

Kilkku, P. "Supravaginal Uterine Amputation vs Hysterectomy: Effects on Coital Frequency and Dyspareunia." *Acta Obstet Gynecol Scand* 1983; 62:141–145.

Kilkku, P, Grönroos, M, Hirvonen, T, Rauramo, L. "Supravaginal Uterine Amputation vs Hysterectomy: Effects on Libido and Orgasm." *Acta Obstet Gynecol Scand* 1983;62:147–152.

Kolata, Gina. "Women and Sex: On This Topic, Science Blushes." *New York Times on the Web.* June 21, 1998.
http://www.nytimes.com/specials/women/nyt98/21kola.html

Laumann, EO, Paik, A, Rosen, R. "Sexual Dysfunction in the United States: Prevalance and Predictors." *JAMA* 1999;281(6):537–544.

Meera, JG, Howe, GR, Rohan, TE. "Nutritional Factors and Endometrial Cancer in Ontario, Canada." Cancer Control, *JMCC* 2000;7(3):288–296.

Mestel, Rosie. "The Science of Passion." *LA Times,* May 1, 2000.

Meston, CM. "Sympathetic Nervous System Activity and Female Sexual Arousal." *Am J Cardiol* 2000;86(2 Suppl 1):30–34.

Morales, A. "Yohimbine in Erectile Dysfunction: The Facts." *Int J Impot Res* 2000; 12(1):S70–74.

Nathorst-Boos, J, van Schoultz, B. "Psychological Reactions and Sexual Life after Hysterectomy with and without Oopherectomy." *Gynecol Obstet Invest* 1992 34:97–101.

Nurnberg, HG, Lauriello, J, Hensley, PL, Parker, LM, Keith, SJ. "Sildenafil for Iatrogenic Serotonergic Antidepressant Medication-Induced Sexual Dysfunction in 4 Patients." *J Clin Psychiatry* 1999;60(1):33–35.

Poad, D, Arnold, EP. "Sexual Function after Pelvic Surgery in Women." *Aust N Z J Obstet Gynaecol* 1994;34:471–474.

Rhodes, JC, Kjerulff, KH, Langenberg, PW, Guzinski, GM. *Hysterectomy and Sexual Functioning.* JAMA 2000;282(20). http://jama.ama-assn.org/issues/v282n20/full/joc81686.html

Rosen, R, Brown, C, Heiman, J, Leiblum, S, Meston, C, Shabsigh, R, Furguson, D, D'Agostine, R, Jr. "The Female Sexual Function Index (FSFI): A Multidimensional Self-Report Instrument for the Assessment of Female Sexual Function." *J Sex Marital Ther* 2000;26(2):191–208.

Rosen, RC, Philips, NA, Gendrano, NC, III, Ferguson, DM. "Oral Phentolamine and Female Sexual Arousal Disorder: A Pilot Study." *J Sex Marital Ther* 1999;25(2):137–144.

Rozenman, D, Janssen, E. "Sexual Function after Hysterectomy" (Letter). *Jama* 2000;283 (17). http://jama.ama-assn.org/issues/v283n17/full/jlt0503-4.html

Shen, WW, Urosevich, Z, Clayton, DO. "Sildenafil in the Treatment of Female Sexual Dysfunction Induced by Selective Seratonin Reuptake Inhibitors." *J Reprod Med* 1999;44(6):535–542.

Siskin, GP, Tublin, ME, Stainken, BF, Dowling, K, Ahn, J, Dolen, EG. "Bilateral Uterine Artery Embolization for the Treatment of Menorrhagia Due to Adenomyosis." At: SCVIR Annual Scientific Meeting; March 2000; San Diego, CA.

Sloan, D. "The Emotional and Psychosexual Aspects of Hysterectomy." *Am J Obstet Gynecol* 1978;131:598–605.

Smith, GD, Frankel, S, Yarnell, J. "Sex and Death: Are They Related? Findings from the Caerphilly Cohort Study." *BMJ* 1997;315:1641–1644.

Thakar, R, Manyonda, I, Stanton, S, Clarkson, P, Robinson, G. "Bladder, Bowel and Sexual Function after Hysterectomy for Benign Conditions." *British Journal of Obstetrics and Gynaecology,* September 1997;104:983–987.

Thomas, JW, Gomez-Jorge, JT, Chang, TC, Jha, RC, Walsh, SM, Spies, JB. "Uterine Fibroid Embolization in Patients with Leiomyomata and Concomitant Adenomyosis: Experience in Thirteen Patients." At: SCVIR Annual Scientific Meeting; March 2000; San Diego, CA.

Toaff, ME. "Adenomyosis." *Alternatives to Hysterectomy.* http://www.netreach.net/~hysterectomyedu/adenomyosis.htm

Utian, WH. "Effect of Hysterectomy, Oopherectomy and Estrogen Therapy on Libido." *Int J Gynaecol Obstet* 1975;13:97–100.

Virtenan, H, Makinen, JI, Kiilholma, PJA. "Conserving the Cervix at Hysterectomy." Letter. *Br J Obstet Gynaecol* 1994;101:587.

Virtanen, H, Makinen, J, Tenho, T, Kiilholma, P, Pitkanen, Y, Hirvonen, T. "Effects of Abdominal Hysterectomy on Urinary and Sexual Symptoms." *Br J Urol* 1993;72:868–872.

Weston, LC. "Hysterectomy Can Have an Impact on Sexuality." *On-Health.* Sep 17, 1998. http://onhealth.com/lifestyle/columnist/item,15017.asp

Zussman, L, et al. "Sexual Response after Hysterectomy-Oophorectomy: Recent Studies and Reconsideration of Psychogenesis." *American Journal of Obstetrics and Gynecology* 1991;40(7):725–729.

Chapter 8 Making a Decision

Agency for Health Care Policy and Research (AHCPR). *Be Informed: Questions to Ask Your Doctor before You Have Surgery.* AHCPR 95-0027, January 1995.

Agency for Health Care Policy and Research (AHCPR). *AHCPR: Improving Health Care Quality Through Research and Education.* AHCPR 99-P007, October 1999.

Agency for Health Care Policy and Research (AHCPR). *Pain Control After Surgery.* AHCPR 92-0021, February 1992.

Agency for Health Care Policy and Research (AHCPR). *Your Guide to Choosing Quality Health Care.* AHCPR 99-0012, December 1998. http://www.ahcpr.gov

Boodman, SG. "Breaking Up With Your Physician: Just As in a Marriage, Problems Leading to a Patient-Doctor 'Divorce' Can be Traced to Communication Difficulties. *LA Times,* May 8, 2000.

Congressional Directory for the 106th Congress: The U.S. Congress Handbook-State Edition. National Committee to Preserve Social Security and Medicare, 2000.

Cooper, J. "Telemedicine, e-Health, & the Law." *Women in Medicine* July/August 2000, 36–42.

Employee Quality Partnership. *How to Choose a Health Plan: A Guide for Employees.* http://www.eqp.org

Fielding. "Changing Medical Practice and Medical Malpractice Claims." *Social Problems* 1995;42(1)38.

Fuchberg. "Countering Spurious Defenses." *Trial* 1994;30(5):28.

Galvotti, C, Richter, DL. "Talking about Hysterectomy: The experiences of Women from Four Cultural Groups." *J Womens Health Gend Based Med* 2000;9 Suppl2:S63–7.

Hall, JA, Roter, DL, Milburn, MA, Daltroy, LH. "Patients' Health as a Predictor of Physician and Patient Behavior in Medical Visits." *Medical Care* 1996;34(12):1205–1218.

Jarrell, RH. "Native American Women and Forced Sterilization 1973–1976." *Caduceus* 1992;8(3):45–58.

Katzenstein, L. "Beyond the Horror Stories, Good News About Managed Care." *NY Times,* June 13, 1999.

Kee, PC, Wong, WN. *The hidden agenda and diagnosis in general practice.* Singapore Med J 1990 Oct;31(5):427–31

Larry, D, Wolfe, S, Lurie, P. "Survey of Doctor Disciplinary Information on State Medical Board websites." *HRG Publication* 1506 (2/2/00) 55 pp. www.citizen.org/hrg/PUBLICATIONS/1506.htm

Liapakis. "The Malpractice Epidemic." *Trial* 1996;32(2)7.

Milligan, BC. "Patient's Rights and sterilizations." *HIS Primary Care Provider* 1993;18(2)36–37.

Mingo, C, Herman, CJ, Jasperse, M. "Women's Stories: Ethnic Variations in Women's Attitudes and Experiences of Menopause, Hysterectomy, and Hormone Replacement Therapy. *J Womens Health Gend Based Med* 2000;9 Suppl 2:S27–38.

O'Keefe, K. "What Is Informed Consent?" *Prairie Law Journal.*
http://prairielaw.com/journal/articles/consent.shtml

Public Citizen, The Health Research Group.
http://www.citizen.org/

The Royal College of Physicians and Surgeons of Canada
Obstetrics and Gynecology Curriculum: Module 3
DISCLOSURE: HYSTERECTOMY
http://rcpsc.medical.org/english/public/bioethics/obgyn_3.htm

The Royal College of Physicians and Surgeons of Canada
Obstetrics and Gynecology Curriculum: Module 10
RESEARCH ETHICS
http://rcpsc.medical.org/english/public/bioethics/obgyn_10.htm

Rubin, AJ. "Texas Is the State of the Art for Law on Patient's Rights." *LA Times,* July 10, 1999.

Steiner, CA, Powe, NR, Anderson, FG, Das, A. "Technology Coverage Decisions by Health Care Plans and Considerations by Medical Directors." *Medical Care* 1997;35:472–489.

The United States District Court
Civil Action Hysterectomy Case
Davis v Hoffman, Puchini, The Reading Hospital
http://www.paed.uscourts.gov/opinions.97D0878P.HTM

Vincent, Young, Phyllips. "Why do People Sue Doctors?" *Lancet* 1994; 343(8913):160098.

Wood, AJJ, Stein, CM, Woosley, R. "Making Medicines Safer: The Need for an Independent Drug Safety Board." *N Engl J Med* 1998;339(25).

Yaron, E, Nelson, PJ, Meier, DE. "Jumping to the Wrong Conclusion." *N Engl J Med* 1998;339(19):1382–1388.

Zuvekas, SH, Weinick, RM. *Changes in Access to Care, 1977–1996: The Role of Health Insurance (99-R054).* Agency for Health Care Policy and Research, 1999.

Chapter 9 Keeping a Journal

HealthAtoZ.com
http://www.healthAtoZ.com

Ryan, MA. "Maintain Your Medical Records." *Today's Chemist at Work* 1999;8(8):49–50, 52–53.
http://pubs.acs.org/hotartcl/tcaw/99/aug/medical.html

Savard, Marie. *The Savard Health Record: A Six-Step System for Managing Your Healthcare.* New York: Time Life, 2000.

Savard, MS, and Forsyth (Contributor). *How to Save Your Own Life: The Savard System for Managing-And Controlling-Your Health Care.* New York: Warner Books, 2000.

Slee, V, Slee, DA, Schmidt, HJ. *The Endangered Medical Record: Ensuring Its Integrity in the Age of Informatics.* Tringa Press, 2000.

Smith, L, Mikkonen, J (Contributor), Hansen, F (Contributor). *Your Personal Medical Symptoms Diary.* M & H Press, 1996.

WebMD. *My Health Record.*
http://my.webmd.com/my_health_record

Conclusion

Bernhard, LA, Harris, CR. "Partner Communication About Hysterectomy." *Health Care for Women International* 1997;18(1):73.

National Kidney and Urologic Diseases Information Klearinghouse (NIDDK). *Prostate Enlargment: Benign Prostatic Hyperplasia.* NIH Publication No. 98-3012. May 1982.
http://niddk.nih.gov/health/urolog/pubs/prostate/index.htm#gland

Sadovsky, R, Dunn, ME. *Patient-Physician Communication on Men's Sexual Health. Primary Care Treatment Updates.* Medical Education Collaborative. 1999.
http://www.medscape.com/Medscape/PrimaryCare/TreatmentUpdate/1999/tu01/public/toc-tu01.html

Sexual Health Network. "Fear of Talking Sex with Docs: Editorial." *Sex Over Forty* 1999;18(2).

Thompson, TL. *Can IR Reduce America's Hysterectomy Rate?* Diagnostic Imaging Women's Health Supplement, April 1998. http://www.dimag.com/db_area/archives/1998/9804whpel.htm

Chat Rooms/Message Boards

Adenomyosis
Host: eGroups
http://www.egroups.com/group/adenomyosis

Adenomyosis Sufferers
Host: Delphi forums
http://www.delphi.com/adenomyosis/start

Black Womens Health
Host: Delphi forums
http://www.delphi.com/bwhhealth/start/

Bladder Buddies Patient Support Group
Host: Delphi Forums
http://www.delphi.com/bladderbuddies/start

Choices (The Hysterectomy Association—UK)
Host: eGroups
http://www.egroups.com/group/choices

Dyspareunia
Host: Inlet Medical Inc.
http://www.inletmedical.org/forum/default.asp

Emboforum—Embolization Support for Japanese Women
Host: eGroups
http://www.egroups.co.jp/group/emboforum

Endometrial Ablation
Host: ezBoard
http://pub10.ezboard.com/bendometrialablationboard

Endometriosis Pavilion Forum
Host: OBGYN.net
http://forums.obgyn.net/endo/

Endometriosissupport
Host: eGroups
http://www.egroups.com/group/endometriosissupport

Endonatural
Host: eGroups
http://www.egroups.com/group/endonatural

EndoUK
Host: eGroups
http://www.egroups.com/group/EndoUK

ERC (Endometriosis Research Center)
Host: eGroups
http://www.egroups.com/group/erc

The Fibroid Place
Host: Delphi Forums
http://www.delphi.com/fibroids/start/

Fibroids—UK/Ireland
Host: SmartGroups.com
http://www.smartgroups.com/groups/fibroids

GYN-ONC
Host: Association of Cancer Online Resources
http://www.acor.org/gyn-onc.html

Hystercity
Host: eGroups
http://www.egroups.com/group/hystercity

Hysterectomy (Men's group/Australia)
Host: The Intradesign Group
http://www.intradesign.com/forums/men_hyst/config.pl?

Hysterectomy Support Forum
Host: Delphi Forums
http://www.delphi.com/hysterectomy/start

Hysterectomy (Women's group/Australia)
Host: The Intradesign Group
http://www.intradesign.com/forums/hyst/config.pl?

HysterPeople
Host: ezBoard
http://pub10.ezboard.com/bhysterpeople

HysterSisters
Host: eGroups
http://www.egroups.com/group/hystersister

Inferendo (infertility & endometriosis)
Host: eGroups
http://www.egroups.com/group/inferendo

Julie's Lupron Page
Host: Delphi Forums
http://www.delphi.com/afterlupron/start

L-M-Sarcoma (Leiomyosarcoma)
Host: Association of Cancer Online Resources
http://listserv.acor.org/archives/l-m-sarcoma.html

Menopause
Host: Delphi Forums
http://www.delphi.com/ab-menopause/start

New Life Changes Menopause Support Group
Host: Delphi Forums
http://www.delphi.com/newlifechanges/start

Sans Uteri Hysterectomy Support Group
Host: The Women's Healthcare Advocacy Service
http://www.findings.net/sans-uteri.html

Surgi-Pausal
Host: eGroups
http://www.egroups.com/group/Surgi-pausal

TeenageEndometriosis
Host: eGroups
http://www.egroups.com/group/TeenageEndometriosis

TTCMyomectomy (Trying to Conceive after Myomectomy)
Host: eGroups
http://www.egroups.com/group/ttcmyomectomy

Uterine Artery Embolization Support Group
Host: eGroups
http://www.egroups.com/group/embo

Uterine Fibroids Research & Support Group (NUFF)
Host: eGroups
http://www.egroups.com/group/uterinefibroids

Uterine Prolapse
Host: Choices for Uterine Prolapse Society, Inc.
http://venus.beseen.com/boardroom/a/25362

Vaginismus
Host: eGroups
http://www.egroups.com/group/vaginismus

WITSENDO
Endometriosis Support Group
http://www.scu.edu.au/sponsored/endo/associations/witsendo.html

Women's Health
Host: Delphi Forums
http://www.delphi.com/ab-womenshealth/start

Women's Health
Host: OBGYN.net
http://forums.obgyn.net/forums/womens-health/

websites

Accreditation Council for Gynecologic Endoscopy (ACGE)
http://www.aagl.com/acgel.htm

Achoo
http://www.achoo.com/main.asp

Adam.com
http://www.adam.com

Aetna U.S. Health Care Policy Bulletin for Uterine Artery Embolization
http://www.aetnausch.com/cpb/data/CPBA0304.html

Agency for Healthcare Research & Quality
http://www.ahcpr.gov/

AJR Newslink
http://ajr.newslink.org/news.html

Alan S. Goldberg's Law, Technology & Change Home Page
http://world.std.com/~goldberg/

Alternative Medicine
http://www.altmedicine.com

American Academy of Family Physicians
http://www.aafp.org/

American Association of Naturopathic Physicians
http://www.naturopathic.org

American Association of Sex Educators, Counselors and Therapists (AASECT)
http://www.aasect.org

American Board of Medical Specialties
http://www.certifieddoctor.org/

American Board of Obstetrics & Gynecology
http://www.abog.org

American College for Advancement in Medicine
http://www.acam.org

American College of Obstetricians & Gynecologists
http://www.acog.com/

American Medical Association
http://www.ama-assn.org

American Medical Women's Association
http://www.amwa-doc.org/

American Nurses Association
http://www.ana.org

American Society for Reproductive Medicine
http://www.asrm.com/

American Society of Anesthesiologists
http://www.asahq.org/

American Society of Clinical Pathologists
http://www.ascp.org

American Telemedicine Association
http://www.atmeda.org

American Thyroid Association
http://www.thyroid.org/

American Urogynecologic Society
http://www.augs.org

Association of Cancer Online Resources (ACOR)
http://www.acor.org

Association of Professors of Gynecology and Obstetrics
http://www.apgo.org/

Canadian Women's Health Network
http://www.cwhn.ca/

Cardiovascular and Interventional Radiology Society of Europe (CIRSE)
http://www.cirse.org/

Center for Complementary & Alternative Medicine (CAM)
Research in Aging and Women's Health
http://cpmcnet.columbia.edu/dept/rosenthal/

The Center for Patient Advocacy
http://www.patientadvocacy.org

Center for Telemedicine Law
http://www.ctl.org/

Clinicaltrials.gov
National Institutes of Health, National Library of Medicine
http://clinicaltrials.gov/ct/gui/c/b

Discovery Health
http://www.discoveryhealth.com

Dr. Koop.com
http://www.drkoop.com

eHealth Insurance
http://www.ehealthinsurance.com

Eldis Health Guide
http://www3.bc.sympatico.ca/me/patientsguide/glossary.htm

Electronic Newsstand (newspapers section)
http://home.worldonline.dk/~knud-sor/en/aviser.html

The Endocrine Society
http://www.endo-society.org/

Endometriosis Association
http://www.EndometriosisAssn.org/

Endometriosis Research Center
http://www.endocenter.org

Female Sexual Function Index
http://www.fsfi-questionnaire.com/default.htm

The Fibroid Zone
http://www.fibroidzone.com

Gay and Lesbian Medical Association
http://www.glma.org/

Georgia Association of Physicians for Human Rights (GAPHR)
http://www.gaphr.org/

Google (search engine)
http://www.google.com

HealthAllies.com
http://www.healthallies.com

HealthAtoZ.com
http://www.healthAtoZ.com

Health Care Choices
http://www.healthcarechoices.org/profile.htm

Health Care Financing Administration
http://hcfa.hhs.gov/

Health Fraud Discussion List
http://www.quackwatch.com/00AboutQuackwatch/discuss.html

HealthGate
http://www.healthgate.com

HealthWindows.com
http://www.healthwindows.com

Health World Online
http://www.healthy.net

His and Her Health
http://www.hisandherhealth.com

HospitalWeb
http://neuro-www.mgh.harvard.edu/hospitalweb.shtml

HysterSisters
http://www.hystersisters.com

Indian Health Service
http://www.his.gov

InteliHealth
http://www.intelihealth.com

The InterNational Council on Infertility Information Dissemination (INCIID)
http://www.inciid.org/

International Urogynecological Association
http://www.iuga.org

International Vegetarian Union
http://www.ivu.org

International Women's Health Coalition
http://www.iwhc.org/

Ivanhoe Broadcast News
http://www.ivanhoe.com/

Quackwatch
http://www.quackwatch.com/

Lesbian Health
http://www.lesbian.org/lesbian-moms/health.html

Lesbian Health (Current Assessment and Directions for the Future)
Institute of Medicine
http://www.nap.edu/html/leshealth/

Lesbian Health Foundation
http://www.lesbianhealthfoundation.org/

Lesbian Health Links
http://www.classicdykes.com/lesbian1.htm

Lesbian Health Web Ring
http://www.geocities.com/HotSprings/Spa/2466/webring.html

Lesbians and Health Care
http://www.suba.com/~leskovec/lesbianhealth/intro.html

Mayo Foundation for Medical Education and Research
http://www.mayohealth.org

MedicalStudent.com
http://www.medicalstudent.com

Mediconsult
http://www.mediconsult.com

Medscape
http://www.medscape.com/

MotherNature.com
http://www.mothernature.com

Museum of Menstruation and Women's Health
http://www.mum.org

National Association of Insurance Commissioners
http://www.naic.org

National Cancer Institute
http://rex.nci.nih.gov/

National Center for Health Statistics (Center for Disease Control)
http://www.cdc.gov/nchs/

National College of Naturopathic Medicine
http://www.ncnm.edu/

National Guideline Clearinghouse
http://www.guideline.gov

National Health Law Program (NheLP)
http://www.healthlaw.org/

National Institute of Environmental Health Sciences (NIEHS)
http://www.niehs.nih.gov/

National Institutes of Health
Office of Research on Women's Health
http://www4.od.nih.gov/orwh/

National Library of Medicine, United States
http://www.nlm.nih.gov/

National Osteoporosis Foundation
http://www.nof.org

National Ovarian Cancer Institute
http://www.ovarian.org

National Uterine Fibroids Foundation
http://www.NUFF.org

National Women's Health Information Center
Online Medical Dictionaries and Journals
http://www.4women.gov/nwhic/references/dictionary.htm

National Women's Health Resource Center
http://www.healthywomen.org/

Native Health Research Database
http://hsx.unm.edu/nhrd/

Network for Excellence in Women's Sexual Health (NEWSHE)
http://www.newshe.com

OBGYN.net
http://www.obgyn.net/

Office of Research on Minority Health, NIH
http://www1.od.nih.gov/ormh/main.html

OnHealth
http://www.onhealth.com

Ovarian Cancer Alliance Canada
http://www.ocac.org

(oxygen)™
http://www.oxygen.com

The Paperboy
http://www.thepaperboy.com/

PatientsGuide.com
http://www3.bc.sympatico.ca/me/patientsguide/glossary.htm

Pleiades Networks: An Internet Resource for Women
http://www.pleiades-net.com/

Polycycstic Ovarian Syndrome Association, Inc.
http://www.pcosupport.org/

Prevention
http://www.healthyideas.com

RESOLVE: The National Infertility Association
http://www.resolve.org/

Rivendell, Enterprise Translation Server
web page Translator
http://rivendel.com/~ric/resources/trex.html

Sexual Health Network
http://www.sexualhealth.com

Society for Cardiovascular and Interventional Radiology
http://www.scvir.org

Society for Gynecologic Oncologists
http://www.sgo.org

Society for Women's Health Research
http://www.womens-health.org/

Thrive Online
http://www.thriveonline.com

U.S. Food and Drug Administration
http://www.fda.gov

Virtual Hospital
http://www.virtualhospital.com

WebMD
http://www.webmd.com

Wellness Web
http://www.wellweb.com/

Women's Health
http://www.pitt.edu/HOME/GHNet/GHWomen.html

Women's Health Alliance
http://www.womenshealthalliance.com/

Women's Health Australia
http://u2.newcastle.edu.au/wha/index.html

Women's Health Initiative
http://www.nhlbi.nih.gov/whi/index.html

Women's Health Interactive
http://www.womens-health.com/

Women's Surgery Group
http://www.womenssurgerygroup.com

WomenWatch, United Nations
http://www.un.org/womenwatch/

Yahoo (search engine)
http://www.yahoo.com

Recommended Books

Ahlgrimm, Marla, Kells, John M. Christine Macgenn. *The HRT Solution: Optimizing Your Hormone Potential.* Garden City Park, NY: Avery Publishing, 1999.

American Medical Women's Association. *American Medical Women's Association Guide to Cancer and Pain Management.* New York: Dell, 1996.

Ameringer, Carl F. *State Medical Boards and the Politics of Public Protection.* Baltimore: John Hopkins University Press, 1999.

Angier, Natalie. *Woman: An Intimate Geography.* Boston: Houghton Mifflin Company, 1999.

Ballweg, ML (ed.), Endometriosis Association, Martin, Dan. *The Endometriosis Sourcebook: The Definitive Guide to Current Treatment Options, the Latest Research, Common Myths About the Disease and Coping Strategies.* Raleigh, NC: NTC/Contemporary Publishing, 1999.

Barber, Sue Ellen. *Hysterectomy: Woman to Woman.* Wilsonville, OR: Bookpartners, Inc., 1997.

Barker, Tara. *The Woman's Book of Orgasms: A Guide to the Ultimate Sexual Pleasure.* New York: Citadel Press, 1998.

Bernstein, Steven (ed.), Fiske, Mary E., McGlynn, Elizabeth A. *Hysterectomy: Indications, Effectiveness, and Risks.* United States Agency for Health Care Policy and Human Services; Santa Monica: Rand Corporation, 1998.

Bernstein, Steven (ed.), Park, Rolla Edward. *Hysterectomy: Ratings of Appropriateness.* United States Agency for Health Care Policy and Human Services; Santa Monica: Rand Corporation, 1998.

Boston Women's Health Book Collective, Jane Pincus (Introduction). *Our Bodies, Ourselves.* New York: Touchstone, 1998.

Carol, Ruth (ed.). *Alternatives for Women With Endometriosis: A Guide by Women for Women.* Chicago: Third Side Press, 1994.

Cloutier-Steele, Lise. *Misinformed Consent.* Shrewsbury, MA: ATL Press, 2001.

Cutler, Winnifred B. *Hysterectomy: Before and After: A Comprehensive Guide to Preventing Preparing for and Maximizing Health After Hysterectomy.* New York: Harper Collins, 1990.

DeCherney, Alan H (ed.), Pernoll, Martin L., (ed.). *Current Obstetric & Gynecologic Diagnosis & Treatment (8th Ed).* New York: McGraw-Hill Professional Publishing, 1996.

Dennerstein, Lorraine, Wood, Carl, Westmore, Ann. *Hysterectomy: New Options and Advances.* Lanham, MD: University Press, 1999.

Dennerstein, Lorraine, Wood, Carl, Burrows, Graham Ham. *Hysterectomy: How to Deal with the Physical and Emotional Aspects.* New York: Oxford University Press, 1983.

Dickson, Anne, Henriques, Nikki. *Hysterectomy—The Positive Recovery Plan.* Out of Print.

Fromer, MJ. *The Endometriosis Survival Guide: Your Guide to the Latest Treatment Options and the Best Coping Strategies.* Oakland, CA: New Harbinger Publications, 1998.

Goldfarb, HA, and Grief, J (Contributor). *The No-Hysterectomy Option: Your Body—Your Choice.* New York: John Wiley & Sons, 1997.

Gralla, Preston. *How the Internet Works: Millennium Edition.* Niedham Heights, MA: Que Education & Training, 1999.

Gralla, Preston. *How Intranets Work.* Emeryville, CA: Ziff-Davis Press, 1996.

Greger, Michael. *Heart Failure: Diary of a Third Year Medical Student.* Self-published, 1999.
http://upalumni.org/medschool

Gross, Amy, Ito, Dee. *Women Talk About Gynecological Surgery: From Diagnosis to Recovery.* New York: Harper Perennial, 1991.

Haas, Adelaide, Puretz, Susan (Contributor). *The Woman's Guide to Hysterectomy: Expectations & Options.* Berkeley, CA: Celestial Arts, 1995.

Heiman, Julia, Lopiccolo, Joseph. *Becoming Orgasmic: A Sexual and Personal Growth Program for Women.* New York: Simon & Schuster, 1988.

Hicks, KM (ed.), et al. *Misdiagnosis: Woman as a Disease.* People's Medical Society, 1994.

Hite, Shere. *The Hite Report: A Nationwide Study of Female Sexuality.* New York: Dell, 1977.

Hudson, Tori. *Women's Encyclopedia of Natural Medicine: Alternative Therapies and Integrative Medicine.* Keats, 1999.

Huff, Darrell. *How to Lie With Statistics.* New York: Norton, 1954.

Huneycutt, Harry C. *All About Hysterectomy: The First Comprehensive Explanation of the Symptoms, the Surgery, the Risks, and the Recovery of This Medical Procedure: With a Special Section for Men Only.* Out of Print.

Hutchins, FL. *The Fibroid Book.* The Fibroid Center, 1998.

Jacobowitz, Ruth S. *150 Most-Asked Questions About Menopause: What Women Really Want to Know.* New York: Morrow, 1996.

Jones, A, Kreps, GL, Phillips, GM. *Communicating with Your Doctor: Getting the Most Out of Health Care.* Cresskill, NJ: Hampton Press, 1995.

Kamen, Betty. *Hormone Replacement Therapy Yes or No? How to Make an Informed Decision About Estrogen, Progesterone, & Other Strategies for Dealing with PMS, Menopause and Osteoporosis.* Novato, CA: Nutrition Encounter, 1996.

Kelley, Kathy P. *Through the Land of Hyster: The Hyster Sisters Guide.* Denton, TX: Ronjon Publications, 1999.

Lark, Susan. *Dr. Susan Lark's Heavy Menstrual Flow & Anemia Self Help Book: Effective Solutions for Premenopause, Bleeding Due to Fibroid Tumors, and Hormonal Imbalances.* Berkeley, CA: Celestial Arts, 1996.

Lark, Susan. *Dr. Susan Lark's the Estrogen Decision Self-Help Book: A Complete Guide for Relief of Menopausal Symptoms Through Hormonal Replacement and Alternatives.* Berkeley, CA: Celestial Arts, 1996.

Lark, Susan. *Fibroid Tumor and Endometriosis Self Help Book.* Berkeley, CA: Celestial Arts, 1995.

Lark, Susan, Herman, Phyllis (ed.). *Natural Treatment of Fibroid Tumors and Endometriosis: Effective Natural Solutions for Relieving the Heavy Bleeding, Cramps and Infertility.* Keats, 1995.

Leape, Lucian L. (ed.), Shiffman, Richard N., Kanouse, David E. *Hysterectomy: Clinical Recommendations and Indications for Use (MR-592/1).* United States Department of Health and Human Services; Santa Monica, CA: Rand Corporation, 1998.

Lee, John R, Hopkins, V, Hanley, J. *What Your Doctor May Not Tell You About Premenopause: Balance Your Hormones and Your Life from Thirty to Fifty.* New York: Warner, 1999.

Lee, John R., Hopkins, V. *What your Doctor May Not Tell You About Menopause: The Breakthrough Book on Natural Progesterone.* New York: Warner, 1996.

Lewis, Jennifer Marie. *Endometriosis—One Woman's Journey.* Glendale, CA: Griffin Publications, 1998.

Liu, CY (ed.). *Laparoscopic Hysterectomy and Pelvic Floor Reconstruction (Minimally Invasive Gynecology Series).* Maloen, MA: Blackwell Science Inc., 1995.

Love, Susan M, Karen, Lindsey (Contributor). *Dr. Susan Love's Hormone Book: Making Informed Choices About Menopause.* New York: Random House, 1998.

Maines, Rachel P. *The Technology of Orgasm: "Hysteria," the Vibrator, and Women's Sexual Satisfaction.* Baltimore: Johns Hopkins University Press, 1999.

Martin, Raquel, Gerstung, Julie (Contributor). *The Estrogen Alternative: Natural Hormone Therapy with Botanical Progesterone.* Rochester, VT: Inner Traditions International Ltd., 1998.

Mears, Jo. *Endometriosis: A Natural Approach.* Ulysses Press, 1998.

Mendelsohn, Robert S. *MalePractice: How Doctors Manipulate Women.* Chicago, IL: Contemporary Books, 1981.

Murray, Michael T. *Premenstrual Syndrome: How You Can Benefit from Diet, Vitamins, Minerals, Herbs and Other Natural Methods.* Rocklin, CA: Prima Publishing, 1997.

Northrup, Christiane. *Women's Bodies, Women's Wisdom: Creating Physical and Emotional Health and Healing.* New York: Doubleday, 1998.

Parker, William H, Parker, Rachel L., Rosenman, Amy E. (Contributor), Rodi, Ingrid A. (Contributor). *A Gynecologist's Second Opinion: The Questions and Answers You Need to Take Charge of Your Health.* New York: Plume, 1996.

Piver, M Steven, Wilder, Gene (Contributor). *Gilda's Disease: Sharing Personal Experiences and a Medical Perspective on Ovarian Cancer.* Amherst, NY: Prometheus Books, 1996.

Plourde, Elizabeth, Plourde, MT. *The Ultimate Rape: What Every Woman Should Know about Hysterectomies and Ovarian Removal.* Irvine, CA: New Voice Publications, 1998.

Public Citizen. *JCAHO; The Failure of "Private" Hospital Regulation.* The Health Research Group, 1996.
http://www.citizen.org/hrg/PUBLICATIONS/jcaho.htm

Public Citizen. *Medical Records: Getting Yours.* The Health Research Group, 1995.
http://www.citizen.org/hrg/PUBLICATIONS/records.htm

Public Citizen. *16,638 Questionable Doctors.* The Health Research Group, 1998.
http://www.questionabledoctors.org/

Rosenfeld, Nancy, Bolen, Dianna W. *Just As Much a Woman: Your Personal Guide to Hysterectomy and Beyond.* Rocklin, CA: Prima Publishing, 1999.

Shandler, Nina. *Estrogen: The Natural Way: Over 250 Easy and Delicious Recipes for Menopause.* New York: Villard Books, 1998.

Simkin, Sandra. *The Case Against Hysterectomy (Pandora Soap Box Series).* London: Rivers Oram Press, 1998.

Stokes, Naomi Miller. *The Castrated Woman: What Your Doctor Won't Tell You About Hysterectomy.* Out of Print.

Strausz, IK. *You Don't Need a Hysterectomy: New and Effective Ways of Avoiding Major Surgery.* Out of Print.

Stringer, NH. *Uterine Fibroids: What Every Woman Needs to Know.* Glenview, IL: Physicians & Scientists Publishing Co., 1996.

Swaney, Arlene. *Health, Happiness & Hormones: One Woman's Journey Towards Health After a Hysterectomy.* Lancaster, PA: Starburst Publications, 1995.

Vliet, Elizabeth Lee. *Screaming To Be Heard: Hormonal Connections Women Suspect and Doctors Ignore.* New York: M. Evans & Co, 1995.

Walters, D Campbell, Quillinan, Edward. *Just Take It Out! The Ethics and Economics of Cesarean Section and Hysterectomy.* Mount Vernon, IL: Topiary Publishing, 1999.

West, Stanley, Dranov, P. *The Hysterectomy Hoax: A Leading Surgeon Explains Why 90 percent of All Hysterectomies Are Unnecessary and Describes All the Treatment Options Available to Every Woman, No Matter What Age.* New York: Main Street Books, Doubleday, 1994.

Index